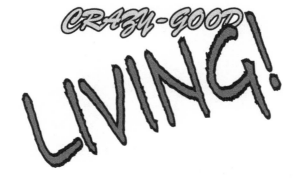

ALVIN H. DANENBERG, DDS

Elektra Press, LLC: Salt Lake City

Requests for permissions should be addressed to Elektra Press, LLC, Rights and Permissions Department, 929 W. Sunset Blvd., Ste. 21-285, Saint George, UT 84770

Printed in the United States of America

Library of Congress Cataloging-in-Publication Data is available on file

ISBN 978-0-9991573-1-2

ACKNOWLEDGMENTS

It all started with my son, Michael Danenberg (www.performance-therapy.com), an Active Release Technique Therapist and a strength training and nutrition coach for over twenty years. He encouraged me to get my act together about nutrition and fitness training. I've also been directed along the way by my various nutrition teachers: John Bagnulo, Kathie Swift, Annie Kay, Jennifer Young, Susan Lord, Lisa Nelson, Mel Sotos, Patrick Hanaway, Jay Lombard, Jim Gordon, Cindy Geyer, Jeanne Wallace, Coco Newton, Mark Hyman, Brenda Davis, Mark Sisson, and Chris Kresser. And, they continue to guide me on my path to wellness. Finally, Faye Swetky and D. J. Herda, who saw something in my writing and encouraged me not to give up.

CONTENTS

PREFACE

In this remarkable, revolutionary approach to treating oral diseases, Dr. Alvin Danenberg advises not only how to cure gingivitis and periodontitis but also to improve debilitating chronic ailments such as coronary heart disease, hypertension, diabetes, arthritis, some forms of cancer, and even excess weight. All too often, a patient receives specialized treatments by medical specialists in their fields, targeting the symptoms of only one disease at a time.

One doctor may prescribe a patient statins for a heart problem; the next may write him a prescription for metformin or insulin for his diabetes; and a third--a dentist--might prescribe for him regular scaling, root planing, and flossing. Meanwhile, the patient ends up entombed in an endless loop of appointments, spiraling medical costs, and additional new symptoms.

At last, *Crazy-Good Living* offers a holistic causative-orientated view that addresses common risk factors. People today eat the wrong foods, exercise rarely, and overload their lifestyles with stress-inducing events. The modern Western diet in particular with its refined carbohydrates, industrialized meat, pro-inflammatory fats, and round-robin of diets robs the body of critical vitamins, minerals, fiber, trace elements, and phytochemicals. The key to detecting such problem areas is periodontitis, which is strongly linked to other chronic diseases. Dr. Danenberg's revolutionary book offers new findings in dental research and represents a totally patient-friendly practical guide to better oral health and total systemic wellness, allowing us to return to a healthier lifestyle and get back to Crazy-Good Living! - Johan Woelber, DDS, University Freiburg Medical Center, Germany

Introduction

Over the course of 2.5 million years, our species evolved into a perfect functioning machine. Dealing with a host of environments and demands, our genetic structure developed the abilities to become the master control center of our well-being. But beginning some 10 thousand years ago, our species has been progressively at odds with our genetic code. In many aspects we have become an unhealthy people. Our modern lifestyles have brought us to the brink of either continuing on a destructive path or taking steps to repair our body.

However, for the most part, we do have control over these missteps. You may be surprised that poor lifestyle choices cause chronic inflammation, which in turn is a major factor in many of today's diseases. But it's true!

Interestingly, almost everything begins with our mouths. Certainly, that includes our source of nourishment. And, our mouths have become unhealthy----more so than ever before in our species' nearly 3-million-year journey. That's why I have chosen to start my story with the mouth. From there, the whole body becomes its playground.

The CDC's National Center for Health Statistics reported from its most recent data that approximately 91% of U.S. adults aged 20–64 had dental decay in permanent teeth. [1] The prevalence increased to 93% for those above 65 years old. [2]

A study published in 2010 demonstrated that 93.9% of adults in the United States had some form of gingivitis, which is inflammation of the gum tissues surrounding the teeth. [3]

Another study published in 2012 showed that 47.2% of the adult population over the age of 30 in the United States had periodontitis (which translated to 64.7 million Americans), and an astounding 70.1% of those over the age of 65 had this disease. [4]

Periodontitis is more serious than gingivitis. Periodontitis is an advanced stage of gum disease where the gums are infected and the bone surrounding the roots of the teeth are breaking down.

This disease leads to bad breath, loose teeth, loss of teeth, sensitive teeth, pain, gum recession, and even spread of infection to other parts of the body.

This is what Pamela McClain, DDS (President of the American Academy of Periodontology at the time of the paper's publication in 2012) had to say: "This is the most accurate picture of periodontal disease in the U.S. adult population we have ever had. For the first time, we now have a precise measure of the prevalence of periodontal disease, and can better understand the true severity and extent of periodontal disease in our country."[5]

So, if you have gum disease or tooth decay, you are not alone.

Obviously, our primal ancestors did not have toothbrushes and did not see a dentist every six months, but they had relatively healthy mouths. They hardly ever had gum disease or tooth decay. Why?

Today, many people see a dentist every six months and also brush and floss daily, but they still have gum disease. How could that be? What we have learned to believe may not be so. Josh Billings (the 19th Century humorist) put it so clearly: "It ain't so much the things we don't know that get us into trouble. It's the things we know that just ain't so."

The why's and how's are related to the nourishment we give ourselves and the lifestyles we lead. As I stated, our modern lifestyle has brought us to the brink of either continuing on a destructive path or taking steps to repair our body. The steps to repair our body are not complicated. The ultimate decision is yours. I'm going to make it understandable, interesting, personal, and easy to get started.

My Lifestyle-Repair Plan is an anti-inflammatory, nutrient-dense diet and lifestyle similar to those of our primal ancestors. My Plan is not a hard-core, black-and-white program. It is a way of eating and a way of living. It is a foundational platform that excludes specific harmful "foods" but allows a vast degree of variation based on one's needs, tastes, and pocket book. It also presents the means to improve your sleep, streamline your exercise program, and effectively reduce your overall stress load, all of which support a healthier *you*. You can use my Plan as the cornerstone to create Your Individual Plan. Later in this book, I offer various tweaks to the Plan to address thirteen specific health concerns that may be of interest to you. And in the book's Appendix, I have included some of my original recipes, along with some variations of popular recipes. These are nutrient-dense, anti-inflammatory dishes you can prepare to help nourish your body. Throughout this book, you will learn that what happens on a cellular level anywhere in the body affects the entire human complexity and how specific foods can help keep your body running smoothly and efficiently.

Before we go on, here is one fact that you need to know up front. Not everything that I discuss in this book has been proven without a shadow of a doubt. Not everything is supported by research that has been published in peer reviewed medical journals. If I were to wait for every fact to be researched by a peer review board, it might take decades before I could make those statements. Most of the information I discuss has been well researched and published in professional journals as referenced in the endnotes, but some of the conclusions I suggest will still need to be researched in a laboratory setting only to be published many years from now.

Who I am

I am a periodontist with over four decades of active patient care. A periodontist is a dentist who has taken a formal postgraduate program of at least three years to become a specialist in the area of gum (more specifically known as periodontal) disease and its related clinical problems. I currently practice periodontics in an office located in South Carolina.

The treatment I perform today for my patients with advanced gum disease is a laser protocol called LANAP® (Laser Assisted New Attachment Procedure). I began using this modality in my practice in 2010. It involves no cutting with a scalpel and no stitches. Patients rarely have any post-op discomfort or swelling or bleeding, and they can go back to their normal routines the next day. With this laser treatment, I am able to destroy the localized bacteria causing gum disease and assist the body in growing new bone around the roots of the affected teeth. But when I started using the laser, I still did not understand the critical relationship between nourishment of the body and gum disease.

In 2013, I started an educational path to learn about real nutrition--the nutrition that allowed our primal ancestors to survive and thrive for 2.5 million years. But, my life-changing journey started years before that.

My life-changing journey[6]

My story is interesting because I could have died.

You would think that a healthcare professional like myself would have learned everything that was necessary to be personally healthy. But, not true. Medical and dental professionals have a paltry amount of nutritional training--and no training in the importance of primal nutrition and lifestyle.

My story begins in December 2006:

I had been in practice for thirty-two years. I was treating my body as well as I thought was appropriate. I ate low fat, high fiber foods including grains, skim milk, fish, and meat. I didn't like non-starchy veggies, but I thought I was doing just fine. I exercised aerobically four to five days a week for about forty minutes a day. One of my loves was to snack on popcorn, which I believed supplied me with healthy fiber.

Then, in December 2006 I had a life-changing event. My daughter (who was staying with me and my wife while her family was transitioning to Portland, OR from Charleston, SC,) was sitting on our living room floor while I was standing with my laptop in my hands. All of a sudden I felt a shock travelling from the computer up my arm. I dropped the computer on my sofa, and my daughter exclaimed, "What's wrong?" I said that I just got a shock from my computer. Her response was, "Dad, don't be so melodramatic." A week later, I had a stroke.

The stroke must have occurred while I was sleeping. When I woke up, my grandson was at our house, and I attempted to ask him if he wanted to go out for breakfast. But, the words could not come out. I was unable to speak. I felt fine, but I couldn't speak. My wife, who is a nurse, realized what was happening, and drove me to the hospital. I was lucky.

My doctors explained that the "shock" that I thought was from my computer was actually a TIA (Transient Ischemic Attack). Many people who have a stroke will experience a TIA days or weeks before the stroke as a warning sign of an impending crisis. I was not aware of such a warning sign, so I paid no attention to it.

While in the hospital for a week, my cardiologist and internist put me on three types of blood pressure meds, a cholesterol med, and an acid reflux med. My vascular surgeon put me on 81mg aspirin and Plavix. Their medical advice was for me to take these meds for the rest of my life. Within three weeks, I was able to speak normally. I returned to work after six weeks.

After my stroke in 2006, I knew that I needed to get educated about good nutrition. So, I began my reeducation. For the next six years, I actively pursued my needed education in nutrition. I thought I was doing well.

In April 2013, I enrolled in a five-day nutrition course that changed my life. I was excited because I believed that this was going to be the program I had searched for to confirm what I was doing currently was correct. I hoped to learn a few new things to hone my skills and update the knowledge that I already acquired. This program wasn't about basic nutrition as I had been learning; it was about primal nutrition--the foods and lifestyles that allowed our species to thrive for 2.5 million years. What I learned in those informative and enlightening five days did change my life. I learned that almost everything I was doing was wrong. That blew me away!

Among other things, I learned that most processed foods were making us sick. I learned that modern grains of any type were one of the worst things I could put in my body. I learned that healthy fats were essential, and anything that was processed to be low-fat or no-fat was unhealthy. I learned that all the fruit I was eating contributed way too much sugar to my body, and leafy greens and other multicolored veggies were required at every meal. I also learned that exercise needed to be efficient, sleep needed to be restorative, various stresses on my body needed to be reduced, and that sitting most of the day was almost as bad as smoking. Wow!

So, I traveled back to my home in Charleston, SC and informed my wife of what I learned. She was not happy. But, she allowed me to make a thirty-day test of my newfangled ideas. We removed all the processed foods, grain products, and sugar aliases from our pantry and fridge, which added up to seven grocery bags that I took to my local Food Bank. We joined our local CSA (Community Supported Agriculture) program to obtain locally grown, organic veggies weekly. The foods we started eating consisted of grass fed beef and wild caught fish; all kinds of shellfish; free range chicken, liver, and eggs; all kinds of vegetables raw and cooked; some deeply colored fruits and occasionally nuts and seeds that we soaked overnight.

At that time in April 2013, my meds were still the same. My HDL was 48, my triglycerides were 120, and my resting blood pressure was 137/87 even with three blood pressure meds. I weighed 184 pounds. My physicians' advice was, "Continue to take your meds." Unfortunately, my physicians were ignorant of the science of primal nutrition and lifestyle, as I believe most physicians are.

As I write this, it's January 2017--forty-six months since beginning an active primal lifestyle in April 2013. I am still practicing periodontics, and I plan to continue treating my patients for the foreseeable future. As I am writing this, my resting blood pressure is 119/72, and my pulse rate is 54. My HDL is 76, and my triglycerides are 78. I weigh 157 pounds. My medications have dropped from seven after I had my stroke to two, which I am currently taking but weaning off of. It has been stated that it takes one month of repairing a nutritionally damaged body for every year of the manifestation of a disease. I am still a work in progress; I have much farther to go to regain optimal health. I am patient, but I am diligent and motivated. I can't believe the way I used to live was slowly destroying me. I can never return to the way it used to be. I am a changed person, and I want to spread the word.

The doctors, whom I depended on in 2006 while I was having a stroke, were exceptional. They saved my life, but I had to learn how to get healthy on my own. I only learned what was going on in my body after I learned about evolution and how our ancestors thrived.

Why didn't my physicians help me understand why I had a stroke, and how I should improve my lifestyle to get healthy? Why didn't my physicians explain how I should wean off my meds over time? The science is there, but most of the medical profession hasn't gotten the message.

While making a change in my life, I also am making a change in my patients' lives. In June of 2014, I received the designation of Certified Functional Medicine Practitioner, which helped me understand why and how diseases start at the cellular level. In September of that year, I received the Certified Primal Health Coach designation, which brought the concepts of primal nutrition and primal lifestyle into a cohesive game plan to incorporate with my active periodontal treatment. In September 2015, I created the Periodontal Module for the College of Integrative Medicine, which offers a 300-hour CIHP (Certified Integrative Healthcare Practitioner) Program for existing healthcare professionals. At that time I was appointed to the College's faculty.

In December 2016, I created and wrote a unique, 5-part, 7-hour CE course for dentists and dental hygienists titled, *Beat the Beast of Dental Disease*. It brought together concepts of primal nutrition and functional medicine together with insights of the development and prevention of dental diseases. Dental professionals now have an evidence-based prevention program they can learn from and that they can teach to their patients.

I teach all my periodontal patients the importance of an anti-inflammatory, nutrient-dense diet and lifestyle. When you enable each cell in the body to function properly by giving it what it needs--which is nutrient-dense real foods and exercise and sleep and reduction in all types of stresses--each cell will help all other cells to thrive. Your gut will become healthier; your overall body will become healthier; and your mouth will become healthier.

I've reenergized my life and reengineered my professional career. I offer the knowledge that I have learned to all my patients and to all who want to listen.

PART I
GETTING STARTED

1. In the Beginning

Everything in life is relative.

When you think about things changing over time, you might compare how things are today related to a time in the past. For example, a gallon of gasoline as I write this costs about $2.20, but a gallon of gas when I started driving in Baltimore in the mid-1960s cost $0.23 a gallon. Styles of clothing have changed, too. And food preparation certainly has changed from when our grandparents were cooking compared to how we cook today. Everything is relative. Some things are better today; some things were better in times gone by.

Old is also relative. After my wife and I moved to Charleston over forty years ago, we were impressed with the city's history and homes that dated back hundreds of years. I thought that was old. Years later, as we traveled to Israel, we saw buildings that were several *thousand* years old.

But even that old isn't *really* that old. *Really old* is when you go back several hundred thousand years and look at evolution.

A change in perspective

When you consider evolution, your perspective changes. Visualize the following:

If you looked out the window of an airplane after boarding, you would see the tarmac and some baggage being loaded into a few planes on the ground--even a few people wandering around. As the plane takes off and begins its ascent, you'd see the tops of some buildings and trees. As you climb higher, you would get a sense of the roads and possible waterways that surround the airport. As you reach the cloud level, you'd see areas of concentrated neighborhoods and forests and geography many miles around. What you'd see from 30,000 feet would be nothing at all like what you'd seen while still on the tarmac. As your visual perspective grew, you learned more of what surrounded that tiny tarmac. What you didn't know existed, you could eventually see. But, how much higher would you need to go to get a bigger and better picture still? A more comprehensive and broader view helps the real story come to life.

When you look at the human condition, the last five or twenty or even one hundred years only tell you so much. To get the real picture, you need to look at evolution. From that perspective you can decipher what has been required for our species to grow strong. Here you may find some truths that have stood the test of time.

When it comes to *truths*, there is only a tiny amount of what we know today to be really true. Some of what we think we know today only gets further tested and disproven a few years down the road. There are some things that we know that we don't know. However, most of the universe of knowledge is composed of what we don't know that we don't know. Perplexing!

Use your imagination

Imagine an animal in the wild--a cute, cuddly little thing. Let's call her "Fuzzy", and let's say she was living 200,000 years ago. In order for Fuzzy to survive and thrive, she needed to chew her food to get the necessary nutrients into her body. As Fuzzy was growing up, something was happening. Her teeth began to decay, and her gums started to bleed. Soon, this furry gal started to have pain when she chewed her food, and eventually her teeth started to get loose. Then her teeth began to rot and fall out. Not only was this happening to her, but also it was happening to most of her brothers and sisters and their offspring. What do you think would happen over time to this animal species?

Unfortunately, the answer is obvious. This species would eventually die off because it could not survive without its teeth to chew the food to get the nutrients that were critical for life. Also, as this animal became weaker from lack of proper nutrition, other predators would take advantage and eat her and her sisters and brothers for dinner. Survival of the fittest!

What did our ancestors know?

The human species has been evolving for 2.5 million years. Over that course of time, our ancestors' bodies slowly adapted to their environments and the foods that were available to them for nutrition. The human body developed a method of using nutrients for growth and survival. It took hundreds of thousands of years for our cells and organs to slowly evolve. Today, we must respect what our bodies need. Our genetic makeup is made up of about 25,000 genes and is 2.5 million years old. Our genes know what they need!

Our primal ancestors were not like the species I referred to above who lost their teeth and died off. As a matter of fact, primal humans hardly ever had tooth decay or gum disease during the 2.5 million years of evolution. Our species survived and thrived with practically all their adult teeth in a healthy state until they died.

It's true that our primal ancestors had a short lifespan of only twenty-five to thirty years. But that's true because the infant mortality rate was very high, and the mortality rate up until the age of fifteen was likewise high due mainly to accidents, infections, and battles with enemies and predators. The number of those early deaths skewed the average lifespan range. However, if an individual reached beyond the age of forty, the average lifespan was significantly higher. These primal beings lived upwards of seventy-two years *without* the ravages of chronic disease.[7]

Obviously, our primal ancestors weren't born with access to toothbrushes and dental floss, and they didn't schedule dental cleanings every six months. Our evolutionary ancestors didn't stop to think about what they ate or what micronutrients or macronutrients were in their food. They just ate, got satisfied, and moved on with the chores of the day. They ate a nutrient-dense diet and had healthy gut bacteria that allowed their teeth to stay healthy. They were physically active much of the day; went to sleep with the setting sun, and rose at dawn. They were social among their clan.

5

Different primal societies of hunter-gatherers ate different foods, as do current day primal societies. But, these foods were nutrient-dense, gathered from their local environments, and allowed their bodies to thrive without the ravages of degenerative diseases.

Then things began to change.

What can skeletons teach us?

I remember going to the Smithsonian Institute in Washington, DC, as a child. My favorite exhibits were the dinosaurs. I was in awe with the age of these beasts. Skeletons told a fascinating story to me as a child.

Today, skeletons still tell the story. Human skeletal remains recently have been discovered in Spain dating back about 400,000 years.[8]

Today, DNA testing can actually look at some dental remains and determine what types of bacteria existed in the mouths of some of our predecessors.[9] Today, we can determine how healthy our evolutionary ancestors were. Science is amazing!

The DNA of the bacteria taken from teeth of most skeletons dating about 20,000 to 10,000 years ago showed a lot of bacteria, but these bacteria were not actively causing disease. In other words, the majority of our primal ancestors had *healthy* bacteria and *minimal* tooth decay or gum disease. Why?

The first evidence of gum disease and tooth decay was documented around 15,000 years ago in an isolated tribe of humans[10]. Why?

Then, from about 10,000 years ago to 150 years ago or so, the bacterial milieu around the teeth from most skulls became unhealthy, and decay and gum disease began to show up regularly.[11] Why?

From 150 years ago to the present, the bacteria went crazy, causing lots of decay and gum disease.[12] Why?

Why were unhealthy bacteria beginning to overtake the dominant, friendly bacteria in our mouths that our species had slowly developed during 2.5 million years of evolution?

At the same time, something was also causing a breakdown in the lining of our intestines. Food particles and bacteria that were never supposed to leak into our blood system began invading our bodies. What was causing these physiological assaults?

Degenerative diseases that had never been part of the human experience began to emerge. Why did humans begin to develop diseases that never were prevalent before?

These are all perplexing questions. Fortunately, science today has provided a number of clues to the answers, and we'll take a look at them in the next chapter.

2. What Went Wrong?

If our primal ancestors ate nutrient-dense foods that allowed them to thrive with no gum disease or tooth decay, then what went wrong?

Today, there is a 47% prevalence of periodontitis among adults in the United States. Periodontitis is the advanced stage of gum disease in which not only the gums are infected, but also the bone surrounding the roots of the teeth. In time, the infected bone can begin to break down. For those who are over sixty-five years old, the prevalence of periodontitis jumps to 70%. When and why did the prevalence of gum disease go from almost 0% to 70%?

It didn't happen in one day. It was progressive and cumulative.

Two and a half million years of evolution brought the human species to a state of high physical and mental development. Functionally, the human body was at its peak performance because the individual cells of the body were functioning as they were meant to function. These healthy cells were nourished by a nutrient-rich diet and stimulated by a physically active lifestyle.

Primal societies did not have the same diets, but they enjoyed nutrient-dense real foods that were available from their environments. However, there was a change in the air. The available nutrient-rich diets were going to become compromised as less nutrient-dense foods became available.

The first documented evidence of gum disease and tooth decay occurred in a tribe around 15,000 years ago in Morocco. These primitive people were eating significant amounts of acorns, which were cooked and loaded with concentrated sugars. The researchers who discovered their skeletal remains suggested that the tooth decay and gum disease were a direct result of the tribe's diet of sticky, high-sugar acorns, which changed the normal bacteria in the mouth to unhealthy types.[13]

A major change began with the emergence of civilization. Civilization allowed people to come together to live. Civilization brought many good things to humans--protection from the elements and protection from their enemies among them. Societies developed farming and agriculture, which brought an abundance of food to feed the masses. Unfortunately, some of the cultivated foods were processed into concentrated (or dense) "acellular" carbohydrates.

"Acellular" means "no cell wall." Acellular carbohydrates had their cell walls broken down and removed. Their nutrient density (the amount of nutrients compared to their total caloric content) was compromised. In time, these acellular carbohydrates began replacing many nutrient-dense foods that used to be the dominant makeup of the human diet.

The timeline for the emergence of these processed foods was about 10,000 years ago that coincided with the advent of agricultural farming. This was the time when skeletal remains began to demonstrate an increasing abundance of unhealthy bacteria developing around the gum-tooth margin.[14] The bacterial changes led to tooth decay and gum disease in the mouth. Dental health was documented to be on a downturn once humans adopted flour and sugars (acellular, unhealthy carbohydrates) into their diets on a regular basis.[15,16]

As the Industrial Revolution took hold around the 1850s, flour and sugar products became dominant in the human diet. The increased and regular ingestion of these acellular carbohydrates significantly increased the virulent bacteria in the mouth and the incidence of dental decay and gum disease.[17]

Healthy carbohydrates are contained in and within the living cells of plants. These carbs are called "cellular" carbohydrates. When these plants are normally cooked, the cell-to-cell links are broken down, but the cell walls surrounding the cells containing most of the healthy carbohydrates are not destroyed. When healthy plants are ingested, the body's digestive system breaks down their cell walls and metabolizes their contents including the healthy, cellular carbohydrates.[18]

Dense, acellular carbohydrates are uncommon in nature. The exceptions are the inner parts of some seeds (including cereal grains) and raw honey. (Raw honey has some unique qualities and benefits, which I describe later.)

Two of the most powerful ways humans created dense, acellular carbohydrates were to isolate and concentrate sugars from plants, and to grind dense seeds into highly compacted flour. In both cases, heat and pressure destroyed the original food's cell walls, resulting in dense carbohydrates. Instead of providing a quick plentiful source of nutrition, these carbohydrates were dead. They didn't spoil over time the way healthy, cellular carbohydrates do; so that made them desirable in people's eyes. But the condensed flour and sugars were innutritious carbohydrates that caused unhealthy changes in the body.

There is a progression of damage that occurs when we eat acellular carbs. Their lack of nutrient density can compromise the human cell's requirements to thrive. The acellular carbohydrates also lead to unhealthy bacterial changes in the mouth and gut as well as damage to the lining of the gut.

Once harmful bacteria are formed and then die, they produce a byproduct called *lipopolysaccharides* or LPSs. LPSs are dead, cellular membranes of gram-negative bacteria, and they are *very* destructive to the body. They can leak into the bloodstream through damage in the layer of the gut lining. Also, they can combine with various unhealthy fats in the gut and can be transported through the cells into the bloodstream. Both of these methods increase the levels of LPSs in the bloodstream. Our immune system reacts to these invaders in the bloodstream and creates cascading events of inflammation, which are highly destructive to many functions of the body. Chronic inflammation leads to increases in degenerative diseases of the whole body.[19]

It was once believed that periodontal disease caused systemic diseases--heart disease.[20] Then the American Heart Association made a statement that there was no evidence indicating a causal link between periodontal disease and heart disease. The AHA suggested independent factors were causing both the diseases independent of one another.[21]

Science now suggests that the frequent ingestion of high-density, acellular carbohydrates in flour and sugar products acts negatively on the human body in several ways. The carbohydrates create a growth of unhealthy bacteria in the mouth and gut that also increases the production of LPSs. This results in damage to the thin cellular lining of the gut. This, in turn, encourages deficiencies in necessary micronutrients that are essential for individual cell function. These unhealthy carbs most likely are the real "root" cause of periodontal disease, cardiovascular diseases, and other chronic diseases of modern humans.[22] Once periodontal disease takes hold, then there may be two sources of chronic systemic inflammation--one from an unhealthy gut and one from unhealthy gums.

I have suggested that the "foods" that produce unhealthy bacteria in the gut also produce unhealthy bacteria in the mouth. In a study published in 2009, a group of ten individuals were instructed not to perform any oral hygiene for a period of four weeks, and they had to eliminate sugars and processed grains and other foods from their diets. At the end of the four-week study, the degree of bleeding gums and periodontal pockets *decreased*. Plaque was present, but the amount of virulent bacteria was reduced.[23] Even though these people didn't clean around their teeth for nearly a month, they had less gum infection. That proved how damaging the consumption of processed-food products is.

The reason is that, when bad bacteria grow out of control, they cause inflammation. In addition to the changes in the mouth and gut lining, these inflammation-promoting microbes change the normal functions of a specific hormone called leptin and other hormones that tell the brain, "I've eaten enough." This communication with the brain is via nerve endings in the gut. If your brain doesn't know you have eaten enough, it won't tell your body to stop eating, which in turn increases the risk of obesity.

Along with eating unhealthy carbohydrates, eating unhealthy fats and oils could increase the inflammatory response. As more acellular carbs are eaten (in the forms of flour and sugar products as well as other processed foods) and less healthy carbs are eaten (in the forms of vegetables and fruits), the risks of obesity and chronic diseases increase. Unhealthy fats bind to lipopolysaccharides in the gut and both are transported directly through the cells into the bloodstream. Even small amounts of flour and sugar are able to produce significant changes. Genetic factors also play a role[24], but diet and environmental factors are more important than genetics.[25]

A different way of eating

Primal societies today eat unprocessed foods, and these societies can thrive on a wide variety of macronutrient ratios (the ratios between fat, protein, and carbohydrate). These societies range from equatorial tribes such as the Kitava of Papua, New Guinea, who consume sixty-five percent of their calories from carbohydrates, to desert tribes such as the !Kung in Africa's Kalahari Desert, who eat large quantities of nuts that are sixty percent fat. What neither of these tribes consumes is carbohydrate-dense, acellular food. These humans rarely have degenerative diseases, tooth decay, or gum disease that plague most modern people today.

Societies leading healthy lifestyles could live into their nineties and beyond. An example is the people on the Greek island of Ikaria, which is located in the middle of the Aegean Sea. There are approximately 8,000 residents who lead a simple, physically active lifestyle, eating nutrient-dense foods gathered from their environment. They essentially are free from chronic diseases. They live a full, healthy life, and then they die. However, when some of them move to other places and adopt different lifestyles and unhealthy eating habits, they succumb to chronic diseases.[26]

Let me take you to another series of islands, The Marshalls, located northeast of Australia and southwest of the Hawaiian

Islands. There is nothing but ocean surrounding these 1,200 islands for 2,000 miles. The largest of these islands is Majuro with 30,000 people. In the early part of the 1900s, the inhabitants of Majuro ate only what the land and ocean provided--various types of seafood, coconuts, bananas, pandan leaves, green leafy vegetables, etc. There was almost no incidence of type 2 diabetes. Then, Majuro became "Westernized" with the introduction of fried foods, canned sugary sodas, donuts, bread, and various other processed foods that replaced their fresh fish, fruits, and veggies. By 2000, seventy years after the introduction of these "foods", 30% of the population ages fifteen through thirty-four had type 2 diabetes, and 90% of people ages thirty-five and older were either prediabetic or had type 2 diabetes. The replacement of nutrient-dense foods with processed, acellular foods caused the spike in this disease.[27]

Here is the good news in all of this. Almost all the damage unhealthy foods have caused can be reversed or at least improved to create a better life going forward.[28] In fact, significant health benefits have been documented in just ten days after switching from a Standard American Diet (a diet high in refined grains, sugar, vegetable oils, processed foods, products from animals fed unnatural foods and chemicals, and dairy products that have been pasteurized and homogenized) to an anti-inflammatory, nutrient-dense diet, which is generally defined as a Paleolithic-type diet.[29] (Throughout the book, I will use the terms *Paleolithic-type* diet or *Paleo-type diet* interchangeably with an *anti-inflammatory* or *nutrient-dense* way of eating.) Even type 2 diabetics may be able to reverse their disease and normalize their insulin production again.[30] The way to do so is to make a lifestyle change by eliminating the unhealthy foods, replacing them with healthier choices and following a more physically active lifestyle.

Eating this way will slowly rebalance the healthy bacteria in your gut and mouth, improve your metabolism, and eventually stabilize your weight. In addition, including stress-reduction techniques, receiving restorative sleep, and performing efficient exercise will enhance overall health. I will discuss all these in more detail later in the book.

So what is a healthy way of eating? Although it is very important to eat the right kind of foods, it is even more important *not* to eat the *wrong* kind of foods. The research suggests that the elimination of dense, acellular carbohydrates can go a long way in creating health and preventing disease. A diet lifestyle that is compatible to primal and contemporary hunter-gatherers is an anti-inflammatory, nutrient-dense diet consisting of animal products from head to tail, vegetables, fruits, nuts, and seeds. With rare exception, these foods have been shown to have a maximum carbohydrate density of around 23%.[31]

So, to answer the original question, "What went wrong?" let's say that our food supply became dominated with dense, acellular carbohydrates that have led to unforeseen damage in the human body.

Calculating carbohydrate density

The term, "carbohydrate density," means the percent of the food mass that consists of carbohydrate minus the fiber component. It is easy to calculate the carbohydrate density of any food. Just divide the grams of carbohydrate in a particular food (excluding the grams of fiber it contains) by the total gram weight of the food to get a percentage. The carbohydrate density increases as more non-fibrous carbs are packed into a given quantity of food. A healthy carbohydrate density is about 23% or less.[32] Eating foods that have a higher density than 23% places more stress on your metabolism and potentially leads to the degenerative diseases of societies eating processed foods. A government Website tells where you can find grams of carbohydrates and grams of fiber in a specific weight of food.[33] To use this site effectively, enter the specific food you are calculating in the space provided on the top of the page and click "GO." Click on the food you desire. Note the Grams of Carbohydrate per 100 grams of food, and note the Grams of Fiber per 100 grams of food.

Subtract the grams of fiber from the grams of carbohydrates to get the non-fibrous grams of carbohydrate per 100 grams of the food. That will be the carbohydrate density of that particular food.

Modern food processing is, unfortunately, very good at boosting carbohydrate density. Here is a list of some foods ranging from low-density to high-density carbohydrates:[34]

Sampling of foods with carbohydrate density ≤ 23% (from lowest to about 23% excluding fiber):

- Chicken, roasted thigh and skin = 0.0%
- Beef = 0.0%
- Lamb = 0.0%
- Pork = 0.0%
- Mackerel = 0.0%
- Eggs, whole poached = 0.7%
- Spinach, raw = 1.4%
- Cauliflower, boiled without salt = 1.8%
- Swiss chard, raw = 2.1%
- Cheese, gouda = 2.2%
- Turnips, raw = 4.6%
- Kale, raw = 5.2%
- Macadamia nuts = 5.2%
- Carrot, raw = 6.8%
- Beets, raw = 6.9%
- Onion, raw = 7.6%
- Honeydew melon, raw = 8.3%
- Orange, raw Florida = 9.1%
- Apple, raw with skin = 11.4%
- Kiwi fruit, raw = 11.7%
- Lentils, boiled = 12.2%
- Leek, raw = 12.4%
- Parsnip, raw = 13.1%
- Black beans, boiled = 15.0%
- Ginger root, raw = 15.8%
- Pistachios, raw = 17.2%
- Buckwheat groats, roasted, cooked = 17.2%

- Sweet potato, baked in skin = 17.4%
- Quinoa, cooked = 18.5%
- White potato, baked in skin = 19.0%
- Brown rice, medium grain cooked = 19.5%
- Wild rice, cooked = 19.5%
- Banana, raw = 20.2%
- 85% Cocoa bar (Alter Eco Dark Blackout) = 22.5%

Sampling of modern foods with carbohydrate density > 23% (from 23% to the highest excluding fiber):

- Cheeseburger, single plain patty and bun = 26.0%
- Cheese pizza = 26.8%
- White rice, medium grain cooked = 28.3%
- Plantains, raw = 29.6%
- Hamburger, single plain patty and bun = 29.9%
- Nachos with cheese = 31.7%
- White bread = 34.7%
- Multigrain bread = 35.9%
- Popcorn, oil-popped microwave = 37.0%
- French fries = 37.6%
- Rye bread = 42.5%
- Bagel, wheat = 44.8%
- Hamburger bun, plain = 48.0%
- Potato chips, plain salted = 50.7%
- Oats = 55.7%
- Granola bar, plain = 59.1%
- Whole wheat hot cereal = 65.7%
- Oat Bran cereal, toasted Quaker Mother's = 66.8%
- Cookies, graham cracker = 74.3%
- Agave syrup = 76.2%
- Pretzels, hard plain salted = 77.0%
- Rice cakes, plain brown rice = 77.3%
- Honey = 82.2%

3. What Your Jaw Is Telling You

For 200,000 years before humans began cultivating grain for consumption, the human jaw and the size of teeth were basically static. However, for the last 10,000 years or so, which coincides with the advent of agricultural farming, the width, length, and shape of the human jaw have been changing slowly while the size of the teeth have remained virtually the same.

So, what is going on?

Although genetics play a role, our environment has been the dominant contributor influencing poor jaw development. There appear to be three major external factors that are affecting the size and shape of our jaws. Two are the results of the onset of agricultural farming, and the more recent factor is the result of how babies are fed. They include:

A decrease in nutrient-dense foods
An increase in soft foods
A decrease in breastfeeding

Decrease in nutrient-dense foods

Nutrient-rich food sources began to decline after agricultural farming provided a significantly increasing proportion of processed foods to our diets. The lack of necessary nutrients in the acellular carbohydrates of these grain and sugar products compromised healthy bone metabolism.[35,36]

Dr. Weston A. Price, a dentist, published *Nutrition and Physical Degeneration* in 1939. In his book, Dr. Price documented numerous observational examples of primitive people who had healthy dentitions and others who had various dental problems including gum disease, tooth decay, and poor jaw development. He identified that those with healthy dentitions generally ate nutrient-dense foods, and those with unhealthy dental conditions regularly consumed diets high in flour, sugar, processed vegetable fats and processed foods. Dr. Price implicated a lack of both fat-soluble vitamins and trace minerals to be the most important deficiencies causing dental problems.

Since then, there have been numerous observations among hunter-gatherers and primal societies who have had relatively healthy bodies with little or no chronic disease. Those societies that continued to eat their natural diets had healthy dentitions, while those who abandoned their traditional diets and began to eat a "Western" diet developed dental problems and even produced offspring with an increasing amount of dental abnormalities.[37]

Increase in soft foods

Soft food sources, which reduced the physical stimuli on the jawbones and muscles of the jaw, increased after agricultural farming.

Processed grains and starchy foods provide a soft diet. Recent research has demonstrated that softer diets create less mechanical stimuli to the muscles and bones of the jaw resulting in a slow decrease in the jaw's density and dimensions over the course of time. Jaws don't need to be as strong or as large if the foods are less hard and less strenuous to chew. Rather than happening over an evolutionary time-scale, the change to the mandible was happening on an individual level as each child was growing up.[38]

Decrease in breastfeeding

Breastfeeding decreased after bottle feeding became commercialized in the 1800s, which had a dramatic effect on the development of the jaw.[39]

Evidence suggests that early humans breastfed until about three or four years of age. In the United States in 2011, 79% of newborn infants started to breastfeed. However, of infants born in 2011, 49% were breastfeeding at six months and only 27% were still breastfeeding at twelve months.[40]

Breastfeeding provides the ideal mechanical stimulation in the mouth for the jaw's normal development. When infants breast-feed, they form a deep attachment to the breast. They open wide and take in enough breast so that the breast is pressing up against their palate. Babies do not merely "suck out" the milk, but instead place their tongue around the breast in a U-shaped pattern. In a wave-like motion they "milk" the breast to receive its nourishment. Two developmental actions take place: (1) a rhythmic action of the tongue "milking" the breast, which presses on the palate, and (2) the subsequent action of swallowing. Both actions play a critical role in proper stimulation and development of the dental arches, palate, jaw, and muscles. As the baby grows, the breast continues to conform to the baby's mouth.[41]

When bottle-feeding replaces breastfeeding, the bottle's unnaturally shaped nipple does not fill or conform to the baby's palate and therefore does not stimulate any widening of the palate to ensure room for future teeth. Also, the infant must create greater suction forces to suck out the milk from the bottle than would be necessary to feed from mother's breast. This forceful action causes the cheeks to draw in, putting pressure on the gums and alveolar bone, affecting the position of the teeth. As the baby grows, the shape of the bottle's nipple doesn't change and cannot adapt to the developing mouth of a growing child, further compromising normal bone and muscle development.

The bottom line

These are observational studies, and there is controversy about the significance of the factors discussed here. But, there is no controversy in this researcher's mind about the fact that eating nutrient-dense foods that represent the nutrition of our primal ancestors will enhance our body's ability to do what it was designed to do. In addition, we should include raw foods as well as crunchy foods like nuts and seeds to stimulate and exercise the muscles and bones of the jaw. We need to chew our food thoroughly. Mothers should breast feed their children for as long as prudent. The Lifestyle-Repair Plan goes into the details of healthy eating and healthy lifestyles. Our health and our children's health are dependent on these primal and natural lifestyles.

4. "All Roads Lead to Rome"

It's a metaphor that has been used since the 1100s, and it means that different paths can take a person to the same place. Concerning the human body, an investigation of nearly all diseases eventually leads to the mouth. The oral cavity is a mirror that reflects many of our body's internal mysteries. What happens on the cellular level frequently works its way to manifest itself in some fashion in the mouth. Many times the signs of systemic diseases appear in the mouth before the systemic disease is even suspected.

Changes in the mouth can take many forms--from bleeding gums to ulcerations in the soft tissues; from swelling of the tongue to changes in the bone structures; from cracking in the lips to variations in color and texture; from loss of taste to difficulty in swallowing; from mouth dryness to excessive saliva. The lips, the corners of the mouth, the soft moist tissues inside the mouth, the teeth, the muscles of the tongue and jaw, and the bone itself are areas that can alter their color, texture, and chemical structure when cellular damage occurs in other parts of the body. What happens in the body almost always will make itself known in the mouth. The mouth is intimately connected to the rest of the body, and the body is intricately connected to what occurs in the mouth. *All roads lead to Rome!*

Here are just a few of the disturbances from various parts of the body that may reveal themselves in and around the mouth:

- Allergic reactions
- Viral infections
- Fungal infections
- Bacterial infections
- Side effects from various medicines
- Blood disorders such as anemia
- Endocrine dysfunctions such as hypothyroidism and diabetes
- Liver dysfunction
- Intestinal diseases such as Crohn's and ulcerative colitis

- Autoimmune diseases such as lupus and Sjogren's syndrome
- Reflux disease (GERD = gastro esophageal reflux disease)
- Bulimia/anorexia
- Stress
- Cancers such as multiple myeloma and leukemia
- Nutritional defects such as vitamin C deficiency and zinc deficiency
- HIV disease

The mouth is not an island unto itself. You must be concerned about anything and everything in the mouth, but many medical professionals often overlook this most basic concept: The mouth is the beginning of the entire subject of nutrition. And the more you know about nutrition, the healthier you'll be!

5. Gum Disease: "What *Me* Worry?"

If certain foods cause gum disease, what's the big deal? Doesn't everyone's gums bleed a little? After all, no one has ever actually *died* from gum disease, right?

Well, my response to the first question is, "It *is* a big deal!" My answer to the second is, "Sadly enough, most people's gums *do* bleed." And my response to the last question is, "Gum disease has been associated with high blood pressure, heart disease, kidney disease, and obesity."[42,43,44]

The fact is that any bleeding from the gums is not healthy. The problem is that most people's gums bleed because most people have some gum disease in today's modern world. So I guess you could say that bleeding gums are normal because most people have some form of gum disease. These bleeding gums are most likely signs of infection, but not always. Bleeding gums may be the first obvious signs of other infections or diseases in the body that one may be unaware of. It is important to have a complete medical examination to determine if there are other health concerns.

Remember what I said earlier: our primal ancestors hardly ever had gum disease.

Gum disease might be the result of the same sources that cause other diseases in the body. Consider this:

Your fingernails are dirty, so you take a nylon bristle brush to clean them. Would you expect to see bleeding at the cuticle? And if you did, would you be concerned? Of course you would!

The cuticle wouldn't bleed unless there was something wrong. Along the same reasoning, the gums around your teeth should *never* bleed when you brush them unless there's something wrong. The gum is sealed around the tooth in a healthy mouth just as the cuticle is sealed around your nail bed. The question is, "Why is the gum seal breaking down?"

But, that's not the only question we face. How about this one: "How will gum disease affect you beyond its indication of an ongoing infection in your body?"

25

There are powerful social consequences of having gum disease, even if a person doesn't know he has this infection. Gum disease can affect a person's love life, his friendships, and even his job security. Gum disease can affect how well a person chews and enjoys foods. Gum disease may affect a person's smile. How? Why? Think about these scenarios:

- Have you ever kissed a person with gum disease? Then you know how it tastes.
- Have you ever spoken to a person with gum disease? Then you know how it smells.
- Have you ever seen a person who has red or swollen gums smile? Then you know how it looks.
- Gum disease can make food taste bad or less enjoyable.
- Gum disease can make a person self-conscious so that he or she avoids smiling.

You may know of someone who has gum disease. You may know of *many* people who have gum disease. But, most people don't know that they have gum disease. Many of those with gum disease only realize they have a problem after their workplace buddies or friends or partners start to avoid being close to them because of the odor. Later, they may notice their gums are swollen or are pulling away from their teeth or their teeth actually are starting to get loose and spaces are forming between them.

The first thing to do if you suspect you have gum disease is to find out for sure. If so, treat it appropriately, and then learn how to prevent its recurrence as I advise in this book. True prevention is much different than just brushing, flossing, and having your teeth cleaned by a dental hygienist a couple times a year. And you'll be amazed at the overall benefits to your whole body when you follow my Lifestyle-Repair Plan.

If you know people who have gum disease but don't know they have it, share this book with them. If you know people who want to gain an overall perspective of achieving a healthier human body, share this book with them. If you know people who want a different approach to the discussion of primal nutrition, share this book with them. And then we can *all* think more seriously about the consequences of dental plaque, saliva, bad breath, and failing health. And take those first critical steps toward correcting them!

6. What Plaque, Saliva, and Bad Breath *Really* Say

When professionals start to think about a healthy mouth and gum system, we invariably start with that Enemy Number One to general oral health, plaque.

Dental plaque

This can be ugly stuff--but not always. When it is thick, it looks like cottage cheese around the gum margin. It can also smell bad. This is the stuff that may create gum disease and dental decay.

Dental plaque[45,46,47] is a biofilm composed of a complex community of salivary components and microbes from as many as 1,400 different species[48], which actually reside in layers and communicate among themselves. There is a healthy state and a pathogenic state.

In the healthy state, both plaque biofilm and adjacent tissues maintain a delicate balance, establishing a harmonious relationship between the two. However, changes occur that transform this *healthy* dental plaque into a *pathogenic* dental plaque. The biological mechanism creating this change is not well understood.

Inflammatory changes throughout the body are transmitted through the saliva and gum fluids and can initiate changes in a cascading way that affect various bacteria either to enhance or diminish their potential for disease. When we eat refined carbohydrates, various bacteria in the biofilm ferment the sugar, produce an abundance of various acids, and demineralize the tooth surface resulting in decay. If there are sufficient nutrients in the saliva, remineralization can occur if the acid level does not drop below a pH of 5.5. Additional inflammatory conditions can alter the bacteria in the biofilm to produce an abundance of strains that initiate gingivitis and later periodontitis.

The first step of plaque formation is the deposition of a sticky substance composed of glycoproteins from the saliva onto the tooth surface, which is called the *pellicle*. Various bacteria begin to attach to this and eventually form a complex, multilayered biofilm. The outer layers of the biofilm are made up of mainly aerobic types (bacteria that live in the presence of oxygen) and the innermost layers are mostly anaerobic (bacteria that live without the presence of oxygen). As the dental plaque migrates under the gum tissues, they turn into primarily anaerobic species. Again, our body's immune system plays a significant role in determining what types of harmful bacteria develop and overgrow. The most aggressive bacterium in periodontitis is *Porphyromonas gingivalis* that actually produces a very potent and destructive byproduct called LPS (lipopolysaccharide).

Research suggests that the bacteria of the gut and the mouth and their inflammatory effects are interrelated and affected by the foods we consume. [49] These effects along with genetic predispositions determine the development and course of disease.

Purpose of saliva

Saliva is a complex, watery/viscous fluid produced by the salivary glands and emptied into the mouth. It provides digestive, protective, and lubricating functions. It has many diverse chemicals to break down foods, protect and remineralize teeth, inhibit precipitation of calcium and phosphate on intact tooth surfaces, promote healing of the oral soft tissues, kill harmful bacteria, and provide an acid buffering effect to prevent sudden changes in acid levels. The flow of saliva increases the most during eating and is reduced to near zero during sleep.

Human saliva is about 98% water. The remaining 2% or so consists of dissolved inorganic ions and organic substances. The enzymes in saliva initiate digestion of starch and fat in the foods we chew. By moistening ingested foods, saliva assists in processing and swallowing our food. Saliva also enhances the taste of foods by dissolving flavorful substances in food and making them more accessible to the taste buds.

It is important to note that saliva inhibits dental decay through the mechanical washing away of bacteria as well as killing harmful bugs. In addition, the high levels of calcium and phosphate ions along with various trace minerals can bathe the enamel surfaces and reverse early stages of demineralization. The important healthy balance easily can be disrupted. By eating fermentable carbohydrates (sugars) and acidic foods, the mouth can be affected immediately.

Among its many functions, saliva contains chemicals that bind to bacteria and destroy them. Unfortunately, serious health issues may occur when saliva is reduced or non-existent.

The healthy benefits from saliva can be negated by unhealthy changes in the gut bacteria, resulting in chronic inflammation.

When saliva is nonexistent

The symptom of dry mouth is called *xerostomia*. Without an adequate flow of saliva, various difficulties can occur: bad breath, increase in decay, increase in mouth infections (including yeast infections, gingivitis, and periodontitis), difficulty in tasting food, and swallowing. Dry mouth can be the result of some medications, damage to the salivary glands, stress, and other systemic diseases that may have an autoimmune component (such as lupus, rheumatoid arthritis, Sjogren's syndrome, and hypothyroidism to name a few). Once again, the gut bacteria play a significant role in the development of autoimmune diseases.

Patients on medications should investigate with their medical doctors if some of these medicines are causing dry mouth and if they could be replaced by other medications. There are some medications that can be prescribed to help stimulate saliva production (such as *pilocarpine* or *cevimeline*). Individuals may find that sipping water frequently, chewing gum that is made with xylitol or stevia, or using a saliva substitute product such as those from Biotene, will reduce the effects of dry mouth. Patients with dry mouth also should abstain from sugar as much as possible, acid drinks, dry and spicy foods, astringents, alcohol, and tobacco. A cool mist humidifier in the bedroom could increase the moisture in the air and might be beneficial during sleep.

Bad breath

Let's face it: Bad breath stinks, and nobody wants stinky breath. But, everybody has had stinky breath or halitosis[50] at times. You may not know that you have stinky breath, but people that come close to you will know. So, what causes it, and what can you do about it?

Documentation of bad breath dates back to 1550 BC when the ancient Egyptians inscribed in the *Ebers Papyrus*[51] (an ancient Egyptian medical document) how to use tablets made from cinnamon, myrrh, and honey to fight bad breath. Unfortunately today, most people still try to mask the odor but never address the actual causes.

Certain bacteria, certain foods, lack of saliva or dry mouth, infections either in the mouth or elsewhere in the body, or stress may cause bad breath. But, the fact is, if you could correct the causes, then your stinky breath would no longer be an annoying problem.

The first major source of halitosis is the mouth, where 90% of all bad breath originates. 80%-90% of this odor from the mouth originates on the back of the upper side of the tongue.[52] This is where many bacteria reside, and where they breakdown dead cells and food particles to form stinky breath.

The next likely place in the mouth for bad breath is located in the crevices where the gum surrounds the necks of teeth and in spaces between the teeth. Bacteria that cause bad breath can accumulate in these hidden places, but more importantly they can cause gum disease, which can contribute to even worse stinky breath.[53]

Other less common sources creating bad breath in the mouth may originate from dental decay; poorly fitting dental work; abscesses and other mouth infections; tobacco; alcohol; dry mouth frequently as a result of some medications; and volatile foodstuffs such as onion, garlic, cabbage, and cauliflower.

The second major source of bad breath is from the nose. This is usually caused by sinus infections and post-nasal drip.

Another source of halitosis can be the odors produced from the metabolism of volatile foodstuffs, which are eventually expelled through the lungs as well as the skin.

Less frequent sources of bad breath are infected tonsils, liver and kidney diseases, carcinoma, lung infections, metabolic disorders, and diabetes.

A likely source that is actively being investigated through peer-reviewed research is the gut bacteria. Healthy bacteria in the gut can be damaged by specific foods, medications, and stress, all of which in turn can affect the bacteria throughout the body. These unhealthy changes in gut bacteria can affect the healthy bacteria in the saliva, which then can change the bacteria in the mouth.[54,55]

Let's examine just how you can find out whether or not you have the insidious infection of gum disease that could be causing mouth odor among *other* damaging things.

7. How To Know if You Have Gum Disease

If your gums bleed when brushing or flossing, you probably have some type of gum disease. But, that's not the whole story. You may have gum disease if your gums *aren't* bleeding because the disease may be deeper under the gum, where bleeding is not so obvious. Sometimes the gums may be swollen or tender, but not always. The teeth may be loose or sensitive, but not always. You may have bad breath or a bad taste in your mouth, but not always.

Gum (or periodontal) diseases are divided between gingivitis, which affects only the gums, and periodontitis, which involves the soft tissue and the tooth-supporting bone. Periodontitis is the more advanced stage. More than sixty-four million Americans have periodontitis, with 70 percent of people 65 years or older having the disease.[56]

When the gum is healthy with no disease, it is sealed around the tooth like a tight turtleneck sweater around your neck or like the cuticle around your fingernail. The gum protects the underlying jawbone that holds your teeth in place.

In gingivitis, the gums usually become red or bleed easily. If the infection moves under the gum, the gum seal breaks down, and the gum separates from around the tooth just like a turtleneck sweater would not stay up around your neck if it lost its elastic band. When this infection begins to damage the underlying bone around the roots of the teeth, the disease becomes known as periodontitis.

Unfortunately, you may have gum disease as I described without the signs and symptoms I mentioned. You may feel as if the gums are healthy because the bleeding you may have had in the past has gone away. You may think that the problem has resolved itself, but the problem just may have gotten deeper without you knowing. As I mentioned, when the gum infection begins to affect the jawbone, it is called periodontitis.

The best way to determine if you have gum disease is to have a dentist or periodontist use a gum ruler (called a periodontal probe) to measure how deep the space is between the surface where the gum surrounds the tooth, and where the gum actually is sealed to the tooth below the surface of the gum margin. This measured space is called a *gum pocket*. Think about a gum pocket similar to a pocket in a jacket. The depth of the gum pocket would be like the distance your hand went into your jacket pocket until the tip of your longest finger stopped where the pocket ended. These measurements are usually taken around every tooth in your mouth, and they should be 1-3 mm in depth in a healthy mouth. Deeper than 5-6 mm could indicate severe periodontitis. The dentist also should check if the gum tissue has receded around any teeth and if the teeth are loose or are being rocked by a grinding or gritting habit.

If you have gum disease, it usually is caused directly by bacteria in the soft film that forms on surfaces of the teeth where the gum tissue meets the tooth. This bacterial film is called *dental plaque*. The bacteria causing the disease can harden under the gum tissue and attach themselves to the roots of the teeth causing an increasing irritant in the area. This is called *calculus or tartar,* and it is similar to barnacles that attach to the bottom of a boat that sits in the water. The irritation from the calculus under the gum on the surface of the root is akin to a splinter deep in your finger that you don't or can't remove.

Also, any habits of grinding or gritting your teeth can make problems worse because these habits wiggle the teeth, which in turn wiggle and weaken the bone that holds the teeth in place.

Some previous dental fillings in your mouth also could cause gum disease. If these fillings are broken down, have rough edges, or don't fit properly in the mouth, they can irritate the gum tissues and harbor clumps of bacteria.

Bacteria, wiggling the teeth from gritting habits, and broken or poorly fitting dental work are the most obvious causes of gum and bone damage. The not-so-obvious underlying problems could be virulent bacteria in your gut; harmful carbohydrates feeding that bacteria; and essential nutrients missing in your diet to help your body fight infection and heal. Any or all of these elements could lead to inflammation--or *worse*. And that's something you need to watch out for!

8. Inflammation

Our bodies are remarkably well equipped to heal themselves. Part of this healing process involves inflammation. When we remove what our bodies do *not* need and give them what they *do* need, our bodies can function as they were meant to function. But when our bodies are exposed for a period of time to these irritants, the result is an exaggerated, chronic inflammatory response.

As an example, if you had an irritant in or around the gum tissues, you would experience an acute inflammatory response. The resulting pain, swelling, and redness around the site of any injury or illness are signs and symptoms of inflammation. Inflammation is essential to our very existence.

The initial response to a pathogen or an injury is called *acute inflammation*. It lasts only a few days or less, and it involves several different biological components, including the vascular system (veins, arteries, capillaries, and such), the immune system, and the cells local to the injury.

The first step in the inflammation process is the damaging of some tissue. After that, pattern recognition receptors (PRR), which are located at the injury site, release various *inflammatory mediators*. Next, vasodilation (or widening of the blood vessels) occurs, which allows increased blood flow to the injury site and makes the site warm and red. The blood carries plasma and leukocytes to the site. The blood vessels become more permeable, and the plasma and leukocytes are allowed to travel through the vessel walls into the injured tissue to do their work by eating up the pathogens.

Emigration of plasma into the tissue results in fluid buildup, which manifests itself through swelling. At the same time, the body releases an inflammatory mediator called bradykinin, which increases sensitivity and pain at the site. This discomfort discourages usage of the injured area so that the tissue has time to heal. All these signs and symptoms of heat, redness, swelling, and pain are necessary for proper healing during this acute stage of inflammation. And, all this is healthy until the causes of inflammation become chronic, and the acute inflammation also becomes chronic. Inflammation isn't meant to be turned-on all the time.

Since acute inflammation causes breakdown of the tissue by targeting damaged tissue and pathogens before building it back up, the inflammatory response has the potential to damage the body over prolonged periods. That's why *chronic*, or persistent, inflammation is so damaging to all the cells and organs of the body.

If there is a constant insult to the body, the inflammatory mediators and their effects are no longer short-lived. The acute inflammatory reaction becomes chronic. There are stressors that induce an acute inflammatory response at first, but then hang around to make the inflammatory response chronic.

Here are some of the stressors to the body that can transform healthy, *acute* inflammation into unhealthy, *chronic* inflammation.

- Irritants and invading pathogens that are not removed create chronic inflammatory responses throughout the body.
- Toxic diets that are high in acellular carbohydrates, sugars, and various components can cause leaky gut and increased inflammation.[57]
- Insufficient omega-3 fatty acid intake has an overall inflammatory response.
- Excessive omega-6 fatty acid intake has an overall inflammatory response.
- Poor sleep habits have been shown to increase chronic inflammation.[58]
- Lack of movement has been demonstrated to increase chronic inflammation.[59,60]
- *Excessive* exercise has been demonstrated to increase chronic inflammation.[61]
- All toxic substances that invade the body can set up chronic inflammatory results.

- Chronic psychological stress can cause hormonal imbalances and chronic inflammation.[62]
- Poor gut health decreases the immune system, encourages *leaky gut*, and increases inflammation.[63]

Not surprisingly, gum disease is a type of inflammation. And, as with all inflammation, it comes in one of two basic flavors: *acute* and *chronic*. Let's take a closer look at what this means to you.

9. Gum Disease: Acute or Chronic?

As we've discussed, *acute* means a condition of short but typically severe duration. *Chronic* means a condition persisting for a long time or constantly recurring.

It would be great to take a pill and have all signs of gum disease disappear. Unfortunately, life doesn't work that way.

When we have an acute problem, conventional medicine is excellent in caring for it. Whether or not it's a broken limb, a heart attack, a severe infection, or any type of life-threatening crisis event, conventional medicine has the means and methods to repair, heal, and save lives. I wouldn't have it any other way. Acute care is best handled by conventional medical procedures.

But *chronic* problems are something else. Chronic diseases don't heal by themselves, and they grow worse over time. A chronic disease usually doesn't have one single cause but rather has several factors that give rise to the disease. Individuals with chronic disease generally have complex symptoms.

Gum disease can be viewed as an acute disease as well as a chronic disease. In its acute phase, bacteria can initiate an infection and inflammation with significant swelling, bleeding, and pain. Taking an antibiotic could relieve the acute symptoms and destroy some of the offending microbes. But, this treatment does not stop the progression of the disease and the eventual destruction of the tissues surrounding the teeth. As a result, the bacteria come back. But bacteria aren't the only factors at work.

There is a chronic component involved with gum disease based on nourishment. "Good" foods do good things; "bad" foods do bad things. The greatest offending foods are the acellular carbohydrates found within processed grain and sugar products. They lack a high density of essential nutrients that are critical for every cell in the body to function efficiently. They have also been implicated in encouraging unhealthy gram-negative bacteria to gain a foothold in the gut as well as increasing unhealthy bacteria in the mouth.[64] These unhealthy bacteria produce byproducts that penetrate into the bloodstream, initiating an inflammatory response, which is a significant factor in activating the immune system and initiating the development of degenerative diseases *everywhere throughout the body*. Bad bacteria in the mouth and a compromised immune system can negatively affect the health of the gum tissue.

In addition, foods containing *antinutrients*, which are compounds that interfere with various processes of digestion, can bind to essential minerals and prevent the intestines from absorbing the nutrients. Some antinutrients can create *holes* in the lining of the gut wall. If our body's cells do not receive their necessary building blocks, our cells will become compromised, further weakening the tissues surrounding the teeth.

To effectively treat gum disease--and, by inference--*all* diseases throughout the body--we must reduce the acute phase and eliminate the microbial, chemical, and mechanical irritants to the tissues around the teeth. Also, healthy food choices and a reduction of exposure to toxic substances from the environment are necessary to enhance the body's ability to become healthier and decrease the potential for future gum disease.

We need to remove all irritants that cause inflammatory responses in the gum tissues. The process of removing these irritants would be analogous to removing a splinter in your finger and cleaning the skin around the area to allow your body to heal itself. Unfortunately, some of these irritants could be the result of faulty or broken-down dental fillings, or fillings that contain materials that are toxic to your system.

By eating and living healthy, we not only improve the health of the gums but also assist the overall body in preventing and dealing with chronic diseases. Remember, primal humans rarely had gum disease or chronic diseases. Similarly, hunter-gatherer societies of today hardly ever have gum disease or chronic diseases unless they move to places where their diets and lifestyles change.

Do you see any connection?

Antibiotics and their role

If a bacterial infection were potentially severe, an appropriate antibiotic very well could be the best and first line of defense. An appropriate antibiotic would kill the bad bacteria, but it would also kill the good bacteria, could damage your gut, and won't generally affect viruses at all. When you factor in the fact that resistant strains of bacteria could develop from the use (or *overuse*) of some antibiotics, you can see why antibiotics may not be all they were once cracked up to be.

There is research that may provide another option to a prescribed antibiotic, although that research isn't yet conclusive. Science shows, though, that essential oils may eventually step up to the plate. Recently, I searched for "antimicrobial effects of essential oils in humans".[65] PubMed is a government site that catalogues all medical research from around the world for easy access by anyone. I discovered a total of 1,035 papers that were published since 1953, of which more than 500 were published since December 2010. It seems as if, despite some controversy, there continues to be a growing interest in researching the power of essential oils.

What are essential oils?

Technically, essential oils are not really oils at all, since they do not contain "lipids." Instead, they are highly complex compounds, which may consist of several hundred different components of alcohols, aldehydes, terpenes, ethers, ketones, phenols, and oxides, many of which may not be known to science. These "oils" are an essential part of plants. They function as the plant's immune system to protect them from microbes and pests that may attack them.

Essential oils have been used in treating human illnesses for thousands of years. In fact, the earliest recorded references can be traced back to 4500 BC. While many have been reported to have beneficial effects, some essential oils have been shown to be toxic.

Today, science has demonstrated antiseptic, anti-inflammatory, antibacterial, antifungal, antiviral, and anti-parasitic properties for a variety of these oils. Specific essential oils also contain vitamins and organic compounds that have been reported to promote homeostasis, which is the state of the body's maintaining a normal range of equilibrium. The purest forms of essential oils are produced through steam distillation and are extremely concentrated. It may take sixteen pounds of fresh plant leaves to produce a single *ounce* of a particular type of essential oil!

How essential oils kill microbes

Scientists speculate that some essential oils produce an exothermic reaction that literally heats up and destroys bacteria, suffocates fungi, and melts the exterior surface of viruses. Some oils may destroy the biofilm surrounding the bacteria, eventually causing the bacteria to rupture. Unlike manufactured antibiotics, microbial resistance to essential oils does not appear to occur, although studies to verify this are still ongoing. Similarly, essential oils used as an antibiotic may kill friendly bacteria, thereby compromising your gut's beneficial microbes.

The potency of essential oils

All these unanswered questions surrounding the benefits and possible drawbacks of essential oils generate controversy. In my research, I found the potency of several essential oils to be comparable to the effects of phenol, which is carbolic acid that is bacteriostatic at concentrations of 0.1–1% and bactericidal/fungicidal at 1–2%. A 5% solution of phenol will kill anthrax spores in forty-eight hours.

In this study[66], if the stated essential oil had a reference number of 1.0, it was equal to the killing power of phenol. Any number above 1.0 indicated the antiseptic power of the essential oil to be greater than that of phenol.

Phenol	1.0
Lavender	1.6
Lemon	2.2
Citral	5.0
Clove	8.0
Thyme	13.0
Oregano	21.0

There are many products on the market, but the formulations are not standardized, which makes evaluating them difficult. Currently, there is no government regulation in this marketplace. Nevertheless, as further research is being conducted, essential oils could be proven to be an effective alternative to traditional antibiotics. Dosing and methods of administration would need to be determined. Regardless, some dentifrices and mouthwashes available on the market today include various essential oils in their formulation. As I stated, essential oils may destroy harmful bugs as well as beneficial ones.

10. Is Gum Disease an Autoimmune Disease?

An autoimmune disease is a disease in which the body produces antibodies that attack its own tissues, leading to the deterioration and, in some cases, the destruction of healthy tissue. Could chronic periodontal disease have many components, one of which is an autoimmune response?[67]

Dr. Alessio Fasano has suggested that autoimmune diseases are a result of these three elements[68]:

A genetic predisposition
An environmental trigger (such as diet or bacteria)
A leaky gut

In his conclusion, if you eliminate any one of these, you could potentially eliminate the autoimmune reaction.

It is interesting to note that many inflammatory markers in patients with periodontal disease are the same ones present in patients with rheumatoid arthritis. [69] Rheumatoid arthritis is considered an autoimmune disease. Some researchers have raised the question, "Which came first, Rheumatoid Arthritis or Periodontal Disease?"

In November 2013, several researchers published a paper demonstrating that specific intestinal bacteria were strongly correlated with newly acquired rheumatoid arthritis in their patient base. Also, these researchers showed that those specific bacteria when placed into the guts of sterile mice caused inflammatory reactions such as those in their RA patients.[70]

It is not a big step to consider that specific unhealthy bacteria in the gut are actually initiating or contributing to the development and progression of chronic periodontal disease. Nor would it be a quantum leap to consider improving the diet to eliminate the offending "foods" that cause unhealthy changes, not only in the gut lining but also in the healthy microbiome of the gut. The lifestyle that may well work the best? It's one I've been using for years now, personally. It's a nutrient-dense diet rich in anti-inflammatory foods I call My Lifestyle-Repair Plan.

Will it work for you? I haven't yet seen it fail anyone who has tried it yet. Will it help you avoid or even heal chronic periodontal disease, as well as chronic inflammation anywhere in your body? Let's find out.

11. Individual Cells and the Roles They Play

Did you know that everything inside your body begins at the cellular level? Don't fret. This isn't going to be a biology lesson. At least, not a formal one followed up by a quiz.

But it's true. The human adult is made up of at least 10 trillion human cells. Recent research has suggested that the number may be closer to 37 trillion.[71] To get a grip on the size of this number, if you lined up all human cells end-to-end, they would circle the earth two times with plenty left over!

Think of a human cell as a chicken egg. The shell of the chicken egg is similar to the membrane of the human cell. The yolk of the egg is like the nucleus of the cell, and the albumen in the egg is the cell's cytoplasm.

Inside the cytoplasm of the human cell, there are little vessels called *mitochondria*, which are critical for the life of the cell. They are like batteries floating in the cytoplasm that produce all the energy the cell needs to do its work. The mitochondria also assist in ridding our body of toxic substances and flushing out old and no longer useful cells.

The evolution of mitochondria is fascinating.

Nearly 1.5 billion years ago, only bacteria roamed the earth. Around that time, a small type of bacteria developed the ability to create energy from oxygen. Larger bacteria engulfed those small bacteria. The small, oxygen-using bacteria created energy for the larger host bacteria. In return, the host bacteria evolved into multicellular organisms, which eventually evolved into animals. The smaller, oxygen-using bacteria that were creating the energy for their host cells eventually became the mitochondria of almost every human cell today. The only human cells that do not have mitochondria are red blood cells, which are also the only human cells that don't have a nucleus.

How important are mitochondria? Think of this: There are more mitochondria in the cytoplasm of cells that require more energy to do what their DNA tells them to do than there are in less energy-needy cells. The energy-needy cells such as those found in the brain, in the heart, and in the retina have approximately 10,000 mitochondria within each single cell!

The DNA (*deoxyribonucleic acid*) is like the script of a play that specifically tells the actors (in this case, the cells) what to say and how to act out their parts. DNA is the genetic script for the entire body, and the entire DNA for each individual resides in every cell's nucleus. DNA conducts the chemistry of life. (There is also a small amount of a unique DNA that resides only in the mitochondria.)

Each individual cell follows its unique subscript that is housed in the DNA and is written only for that particular cell. That way, a muscle cell acts only as a muscle cell; a brain cell acts only as a brain cell; and a gum-tissue cell acts only as a gum-tissue cell.

The mitochondria, which provide the energy for all these cells, are also hungry. If they do not get all the required B vitamins, minerals, antioxidants, and healthy fats (including saturated fats, omega 3 fatty acids, and omega 6 fatty acids), they will not function properly.

Compare mitochondria cells to a flashlight. If the battery is strong, the light shines brightly. If the battery is weak, the light becomes dimmer, even though it may still work. The weak flashlight just doesn't live up to the standards expected of it. But if you replace that weak battery with a fresh one, the flashlight will function as it did when it was brand new.

And so, too, is it with the body's individual cells. If their mitochondria are not firing on all cylinders, they may function, but their ability to do what they were designed to do for the cell will be compromised. Mitochondria must be kept fresh for peak performance.

Cell talk

All cells use hormones to talk to one another through biochemical processes. Hormones attach to the membranes of cells and transmit critical information into the cells. Hormones can tell cells to speed up and work harder at what they do, or hormones can tell cells to slow down. Cells obtain their food to function properly by absorbing nutrients through their membranes.

The building blocks for each cell as well as all of its mitochondria are made up of many types of nutrients that are ultimately derived from the foods we eat. If the quality of the food is inferior, the cell may function but at a subpar level, as with the flashlight with the weak batteries. If the batteries die, the flashlight dies. If the mitochondria die, the cell dies.

Our environment--which includes the food we eat--enters the picture by actually *turning on* or *turning off* specific genes. For example, if you had a gene that might increase your risk of cancer, that gene could be made to *turn off* its biological function through the chemistry found in the food you eat and in the lifestyle you lead. This science is called *epigenetics*. The concept of epigenetics is similar to a director dictating how the actors should perform.

Carrying that analogy one step further, think of the human life span as a stage play. The individual human cells are the actors in this play. The DNA within each cell provide the script, telling each actor how to do what he is cast to do. The structure of the DNA functions as the words of the script, and the genes are specific phrases in the script that define important actions or events that are designed to take place. While the script essentially remains the same, the director of the play is free to choose to change some of these specific phrases, thus altering the play. In other words, through epigenetics, the director can affect the performance of certain genes.

Because of epigenetics, people get sick due to their vulnerable genes interacting with various factors in the environment. Our bodies can turn genes "off" and they can turn genes "on." In fact, 90% of chronic disease is driven by the environment and not by our genes. [72] There is an abundant body of scientific research confirming that toxicity and deficiency cause disease. We are

53

exposed to toxic substances that accumulate in our system, and we don't get what we need to survive.[73]

Practically all diseases can be traced back to problems on a cellular level, and they almost all look alike on that level. Too many free radicals affecting the health of their mitochondria, too many accumulated toxic substances, and too much inflammation are all factors creating cell dysfunction and chronic disease. All these problems can evolve from what we put, or *don't* put, into our bodies.

To break out of the health trap in which many of us are entwined, we need to avoid toxic substances that get into our bodies, and we need to ingest the foods that our bodies are designed to use for growth and energy. Avoiding toxic substances means buying foods that are not contaminated with fertilizers and hormones and are free of preservatives and other artificial additives. Getting the right food consists of eating fresh vegetables, fruit, nuts, seeds, and pasture-raised or wild-caught animal products from nose to tail.

Why is all this important? If cells do not communicate effectively or if they are not fed adequately, they will not be able to do what the body needs them to do. If the cell were a liver cell, it might not be able to help remove toxic substances from the body; if it were a brain cell, it might not be able to remember important facts; if it were a cell in the pancreas, it might not be able to produce adequate insulin; if it were an immune cell in the gum tissue, it might not be able to defend the area from a gum infection. Each cell is specialized to function in some way that eventually allows the whole, complex body to be the best it can be. When cells malfunction, then organs malfunction. When organs malfunction, then *you* malfunction.

The bottom line is this: the quality of the food we eat and the lifestyle we live are critical for the health of each cell, which becomes critical for the function of the whole body, which becomes crucial to maintaining a healthy mouth. Most importantly, even though each of us has genes that may create a specific outcome in life, because of epigenetics, our food choices and lifestyle choices have more influence on who we are than our genes.

But what if individual cells are not functioning properly? Conventional medicine does not do a good job in identifying disease on a cellular level. Is there a form of medicine that *can* deal with cellular dysfunction?

Yes, there is, and we'll learn all about it in the next chapter.

12. Functional Medicine

How often do you have a headache and reach for an aspirin or other pain reliever? How often do you have a stuffy nose and reach for an antihistamine? We live in a society that wants a pill for every ill. When we go to the doctor, most of us want a prescription to rid us of what ails us. How often does our medical doctor look for the underlying cause to treat a problem instead of prescribing a medication just to reduce the symptoms we're experiencing?

Many of us have come to know that much of medicine today is concerned with treating the *symptoms* of a disease. Thousands of names have been created to label these disease entities along with their symptoms. And thousands of prescription medicines and over-the-counter supplements have been developed to treat their individual symptoms. And then there are medicines to treat the side effects of the original medicines. It is often a frustrating battle.

Is there another standard? Is there a way to identify why cells in our body function poorly? Is there a process to rectify the breakdown in communication between cells so healing could occur? Is there a science that treats the underlying causes, and not just the symptoms, of disease?

Well, the answer is *yes*. The science is called *Functional Medicine*. Functional Medicine looks for the cause of cellular miscommunication.

Thomas Edison is credited with saying, "The doctor of the future will give no medicine, but will interest his patients in the care of the human frame, in a proper diet, and in the cause and prevention of disease."

When we eat certain harmful "foods" (like dense acellular carbohydrates), the bad bacteria in the gut overpopulate, increasing the unhealthy bacteria in the mouth. These harmful food products weaken our gut lining, which is only one cell-layer thick. This protective lining is the primary physical barrier that separates the outside world from our inner self. Bacterial byproducts and undigested proteins accumulating in our gut are able to leak into our blood. This portal to our blood system allows a vicious chain of events to occur, affecting our bodily functions. Then, a host of degenerative diseases have a chance to simmer and develop--sometimes over many years. Along with these changes, the bacteria in our mouths become more virulent, which form the dental plaque that can initiate gum disease. From gum disease, infection can leak into the blood system and affect other organs.

Nearly all chronic diseases share mitochondrial dysfunction, excessive inflammation, high cortisol levels, and other markers of broken biochemistry and incorrect communication within and between our cells. If removing local irritants that are causing gum disease, improving nourishment, and helping our body flush out the toxic substances are ineffective, then functional medicine could delve deeper into more obscure underlying causes.

Functional medicine looks at various tests including blood, saliva, and stool in order to help pinpoint the physiological processes that are out of balance and repair them. However, repair will take time. Although our cells are in a constant state of repair by replacing tissues with fresh ones, it is not performed at the same rate.

The lining of the gut from the mouth to the anus is replaced every couple of weeks. The skin cells are replaced about once a year. The liver and kidney cells are replaced about every 1-3 years. Cells of blood vessels are replaced about every 3 years. Brain cells about every 7 years; heart muscle cells about every 7-10 years; and skeletal cells about every 10 years.[74] Obviously, the gut lining is by far the most active!

Applying the concepts of nutrient-dense foods, we could begin to heal our gut, which could begin a healing process for our mouths as well as the rest of our body. In addition, removing the irritants and toxic substances accumulated in our body and avoiding exposure to environmental toxic substances will also improve the healing process. If there is continuing cellular dysfunction, *Functional Medicine* could determine the sources and recommend means of repair.

Several organizations provide education and certification for healthcare professionals in functional medicine. A few examples: College of Integrative Medicine [75], Institute for Functional Medicine[76], and Functional Medicine University[77]. Their websites might provide names of practitioners in your area for consultation and necessary treatment.

Functional medicine identifies cellular dysfunction, but for cells to work the way they were meant to, they need to be fed the necessary nutrients to survive and thrive. But in order for the food you eat to become the fuel for the cells, it needs to go through your body's digestive system. So let's take a closer look at just how that process works.

13. A Tour Down the Alimentary Canal

In Part II of this book, I discuss the food choices you can make to obtain the nourishment to help you survive and thrive. These foods will provide the nutrient sources for every cell in your body. But first, it might be interesting to know how this nourishment gets from the *outside of you* to the *inside of you* in order to do so many miraculous things. So, let's take a tour of the alimentary canal, the route to healthy nourishment.

In the human body, everything begins with your mouth. That's where the digestive system begins and continues on a circuitous pathway for a distance of nearly thirty feet until it ends with your anus. In a nutritionally healthy individual, the time for food to travel, be digested, be absorbed, and be ready for its exit is between twelve and twenty-four hours. There are many stops along the way where important functions occur. In addition, there are several organs that participate in the digestion of your food and that connect in some way to this long, meandering "food tube."

The tube is called the alimentary canal, or the gastrointestinal tract. This passage is made up of the oral cavity, pharynx, esophagus, stomach, small intestine, and large intestine ending with the rectum and anus. What enters through your mouth should never get into your bloodstream until the elements are broken down sufficiently enough to be allowed admittance into your body. This tube from your mouth to your anus houses the "outside world." The only structure protecting the "inside of you" from this "outside of you" is a thin layer of biologically active but vulnerable gut cells that are home for an enormous number and varieties of microbes.

Other important organs that help your body to digest food include the teeth, tongue, salivary glands, liver, gallbladder, and pancreas.

The variety of microbes in the intestines, called the *gut microbiome*, are considered a separate organ. Your body is made up of ten times more microbial cells than human cells! The question to think about is this: *Are we a human body living with bacteria, or are we bacteria living within a human body?*

The oral cavity

The real digestion process starts when you think about and smell food, both activities that begin the flow of the gastric juices within your body. But the mechanical process actually begins when you place food in your mouth. Your teeth start chopping the food into small pieces, and the saliva that is produced by three separate salivary glands helps moisten the food. Saliva also contains an enzyme called amylase that begins to break down starch. Then the tongue and other muscles push the food into the pharynx.

Pharynx

The pharynx (Greek for "throat") is a cone-shaped passageway leading from the oral and nasal cavities in the head to the esophagus and larynx. The pharynx contains both circular and longitudinal muscles. The circular muscles form constrictions that help push food to the esophagus while preventing air from being swallowed, while the longitudinal fibers lift the walls of the pharynx during the act of swallowing.

Esophagus

The esophagus is a muscular tube connecting the pharynx to the stomach where the chewed food continues along its path down and out. The average pH in the esophagus is 7.0, which is neutral. A series of muscular contractions, called *peristalsis*, takes over to transport the food through the rest of the system. At the end of the esophagus is a muscular ring called the *lower esophageal sphincter* or *cardiac sphincter*. The function of this sphincter is to close the end of the esophagus and trap food in the stomach so that it does not move back up into the esophagus.

Stomach

The next stop along the journey is the stomach, which is a muscular bag that acts as a storage tank for food so that the body has time to digest large meals properly. The stomach's gastric juice, which is primarily a mix of hydrochloric acid and a digestive enzyme called *pepsin*, starts breaking down proteins and killing potentially harmful bacteria. The pH of a healthy stomach is between 1.0 and 3.0, which is *very* acidic. Absorption begins in the stomach with simple molecules such as water and alcohol being passed directly into the bloodstream. After an hour or two of this process, a thick semi-liquid paste called *chyme* forms. At this point the pyloric sphincter valve opens and the chyme enters the first part of the small intestine.

Small intestine

The small intestine, which is about twenty feet long, is coiled like a hose. Its inside surface is full of numerous ridges and folds that resemble a shag rug. These folds are used to maximize the digestion of food and to absorb nutrients.

The small intestine is made up of three sections: the first part is the *duodenum*; the middle section is called the *jejunum*; and the last part is called the *ileum*. The pH of the duodenum rises from the naturally acidic range of 1.0 to 3.0 of the stomach to a range of 4.0 - 5.0. Then in the lower part of the small intestine (jejunum and ileum), the pH rises again to a range of 6.5 - 7.5.

The duodenum is the shortest segment of the small intestine. It receives the chyme from the stomach and plays a vital role in the chemical digestion of this food mass in preparation for absorption in the small intestine. Many chemical secretions from the pancreas, liver, and gallbladder mix with the chyme in the duodenum to assist digestion. By the time food has left the duodenum, most has been reduced to its chemical building blocks--fatty acids, amino acids, monosaccharides, and nucleotides.

The bulk of chemical digestion takes place in the duodenum because of the action of the pancreas. The pancreas secretes an incredibly strong digestive cocktail known as pancreatic juice, which is capable of digesting lipids, carbohydrates, proteins, and nucleic acids. The pancreas delivers its digestive juices to the duodenum through small tubes called ducts.

The liver's main function in digestion is the production of bile and its secretion into the duodenum. Bile is used to mechanically break fats into smaller globules.

The gallbladder is another important organ in digestion and is used to store and recycle excess bile from the small intestine so that it can be reused for the digestion of subsequent meals. The gallbladder squeezes bile through the bile ducts, which connect the gallbladder and liver to the duodenum. The bile mixes with the fat in food in the duodenum. The bile acids dissolve fat into a water-soluble mixture in the intestine, much the way dish detergents dissolve fats from a greasy frying pan. This allows the intestinal and pancreatic enzymes to digest the fat molecules.

Friendly bacteria in the small intestine also produce some of the enzymes needed to digest carbohydrates.

The small intestine absorbs almost 90% of the digested food molecules and minerals, as well as some water. All this happens through the small intestine's single cell-layer-thick lining that separates the outside world from your bloodstream.

These absorbed nutrients are then transported to the liver through the hepatic portal vein. The liver is responsible for metabolizing the elements of carbohydrates, lipids, and proteins into biologically useful materials. The liver also breaks down toxic substances and unwanted chemicals, such as alcohol, which are detoxified and passed from the body as waste.

Whatever material is left in the small intestine goes into the large intestine.

Large intestine

The large intestine is about five feet long. It wraps around the upper and side borders of the small intestine. The pH in the large intestine drops from a range of 6.5 to 7.5 in the lower part of the small intestine to a slightly more acidic range of 5.6 - 6.9.

Basically, the large intestine absorbs water and vitamins B and K. It contains many healthy bacteria that aid in the breakdown of wastes while extracting some nutrients. The final product that ends this trip down the alimentary canal is the waste product called feces, which is stored in the rectum and exits the body--finally!--through the anus.

14. Just My Gut Feeling

More than 2,000 years ago, Hippocrates said, "All disease begins in the gut." Only now has science begun to understand the real meaning and accuracy of that statement. Research over the past two decades has revealed that gut health is critical to overall health and that an unhealthy gut contributes to a wide range of diseases, including gum diseases, diabetes, obesity, rheumatoid arthritis, autism spectrum disorder, depression, chronic fatigue syndrome, and other maladies and autoimmune diseases.

In fact, many researchers believe that supporting intestinal health and restoring the integrity of the gut barrier will be one of the most important areas of concern for medicine going forward. Since the year 2000, published articles on the gut microbiome have increased more than tenfold.

It turns out that your gut isn't merely a tube where food starts and ends. You are more than what you eat; you are what you *absorb*. The total trip from end to end normally takes from twelve to twenty-four hours in an adult who is nutritionally healthy. Whatever affects that trip down the canal can affect overall health.

The following discussion describes your "second brain," the gut microbiota, and the gut barrier.

The second brain

There is an extensive network of neurons located between the muscular layers in the walls of the digestive system. Believe it or not, these neurons actually have the same structure as the neurons of the brain! Both produce similar chemicals called neurotransmitters and hormones. They talk to cells and tell them what to do. These neurons in the gut are called the *enteric nervous system*, about which Dr. Michael Gershon wrote a groundbreaking book called *The Second Brain*[78].

The neurotransmitters (such as acetylcholine, dopamine, and serotonin) that are produced in our brain are also produced in our gut. These chemicals regulate our emotional and psychological well-being. Dr. Gershon determined that 90% of the "feel good" neurotransmitter, serotonin, is produced and stored in the intestinal walls where it regulates peristalsis and sensory transmissions. Not too long ago, researchers thought that the brain regulates the gut. Now we know that the communication actually goes both ways to and from the gut. Here are some effects of this two-way communication system:

- You have a big test coming up in school and you're understandably nervous. You might get diarrhea or might vomit from the fear of taking the test.
- You may be overly depressed about something, and you go crazy with binging on junk food. The uncontrollable eating of unhealthy carbohydrates leads to a rapid release of chemicals and hormones from both "brains" that stimulate your feeling of well-being.
- Your stomach "feels bad," making it difficult for you to think clearly.
- You get constipated and feel bloated, and you don't feel like being with people.
- You have a good bowel movement in the morning, and you feel great for the rest of the day.
- When you gently massage a baby's belly, the baby suddenly grows mellow.

The reasons behind all these reactions stem partly from the brain and partly from the gut.

Gut microbiome

Can you imagine counting from *one* to a *million*? If you counted really fast, running off five numbers a second, it would take you 55.56 hours nonstop! Can you imagine counting to 10 *trillion*? When written, the number looks like this: 10,000,000,000,000. When counted out loud, you'd need more than 63,000 years to complete your task!

The average adult is made up of more than 10 trillion human cells. But, the average adult is a host for over 100 trillion microbes that inhabit our body, 70% of which inhabit the large intestine.

That's ten times the number of human cells that make us who we are. An analysis involving multiple subjects has suggested that the collective human gut microbiota is composed of over 35,000 different bacterial species[79]. We are more microbes than human! Most of these microbes live in our gut and provide a tremendous benefit to us.

We are not aware that these bacteria coexist with us. Many microbes, good and bad, can be destroyed through the use of antibiotics or even during severe diarrhea. The gut microbes also don't like many drugs or toxic substances that are continuously bombarding their lifestyle. Yet, their function is critical to our ability to survive and thrive. A healthy gut microbiome also is critical for a healthy mouth.

Healthy bacteria make vitamins and other nutrients, and they affect our immune system. They enhance the digestion of our food and our total health when they populate our guts in proper ratios, varieties of species, and numbers. They specifically nourish the cells that line the gut and provide a first line of defense against invaders into the body. A recent study demonstrated that the gut microbiome also might influence the health of the blood brain barrier.[80] When the ratios of unhealthy to healthy bacteria soar, overall health is compromised. When the gut microbiome falls out of balance and the "bad guys" proliferate, the imbalance is called *dysbiosis*. The byproducts of bad bacteria are toxic and inflammatory to the body and destructive to the cells lining the gut.

Yeast cells (the fungal strains of microbes) are also damaging in disproportionate numbers. They love to eat sugars and other fermentable carbohydrates. But their byproducts cause damage to the gut lining while creating gas and bloating.

The life of our gut microbes started at our birth. Prior to that time, our guts were essentially sterile. Then passage through the birth canal inoculated our gut with our mother's healthy microbes. If we were born through caesarian section, then our first inoculation of microbes that would populate our gut would come from the immediate environment surrounding the birth. Breastfeeding and other forms of nourishment in the first months of life continue to influence the gut microbiome. At around three years of age, our gut microbiome is mostly fixed for the rest of our lives. When we reach our senior years, the gut microbiota begin to differ from both the core microbiota and the diversity levels we previously hosted.

So, where are the microbes found in this intestinal tube? They find their home in various places throughout the alimentary canal. The mouth, pharynx, and esophagus are hosts to many forms of microbes. Almost no bacteria live in the highly acidic stomach. Even though the acid level in the duodenum is lower, few bacteria live there, either, because of the hostile reaction to bile and pancreatic juices. The rest of the small intestine can host more bacteria, but by far the greatest majority of microbes reside in the large intestine.

Most of the bacteria in the gut live in a mucus layer that lines the intestines. Some bacteria and their offspring are permanent residents of this mucus layer while others simply pass through the intestinal tract mixing with the remnants of our food. The proper ratios, numbers, and varieties of good microbes to bad dictate the health of the gut.

When we ingest foods that contain live bacteria, such as yogurt, kefir, sauerkraut, and even probiotic capsules, these become the transient bacteria as they pass through the canal. They can assist and support our resident healthy microbiome. When we eat foods that disturb homeostasis in our gut microbes; or when we experience physical, chemical, or emotional stresses of any type, the result can lead to dysbiosis.

So, in short, our gut microbiome:

- Produces short-chain fatty acids[81].
- Produces acetic acid and propanoic acid[82]
- Ferments carbohydrates[83]
- Synthesizes essential nutrients[84]

- Helps metabolize bile acids and cholesterol[85]
- Supports healthy gut lining[86]
- Assists the immune system[87]

Interestingly, bad bacteria don't *always* cause obvious symptoms in the gut. Frequently, damage to the gut lining can cause symptoms that are well removed from their source. One such example is lesions in the mouth. However, *some* gut symptoms resulting from an excess of bad microbes include:

- Bloating
- Gas
- Dark and foul-smelling feces
- Constipation
- Irritable colon
- Diverticulitis
- Polyps
- Crohn's disease
- Colon cancer, etc.

The short turnover time of gut cells of every one to two weeks helps maintain homeostasis of the gut microbiome. However, overpopulation of bad bacteria over a long period of time can lead to a breakdown in the cell lining of the gut, allowing leakage into the bloodstream.

Gut barrier

Think of the lining of your digestive tract as a fine mesh net with extremely small holes that allow only specific substances of a specific size to pass through. If the substances are smaller than the holes in the net, they can pass through. If the substances are larger than the holes, they can't. These bigger particles remain in the gut until they're broken down into their smaller basic elements. Only *then* can they pass out of the gut. This is how a healthy gut should function. Your gut lining works as a barrier keeping out those bigger particles that can damage your system.

If the "fine mesh net" in your digestive tract gets damaged and bigger holes develop, some of these not fully digested food particles could pass through into your bloodstream. This is called a *leaky gut*, or more specifically *increased intestinal permeability*. Some of the larger particles that should never seep through are able to penetrate. These undigested substances might include proteins (such as gluten that is not able to be completely digested by the human gut), bad bacteria along with their harmful byproducts, and food particles that have not been broken down into their biologically effective components. Toxic waste could also leak from the inside of the intestinal wall into the bloodstream. All substances that leak into the bloodstream can initiate inflammatory, along with autoimmune, responses, all of which can manifest themselves throughout the body--including the mouth. Dr. Alessio Fasano has researched and eloquently described the elements leading to a leaky gut.[88]

- Poor diet
- Bacterial imbalance
- Chronic stress
- Toxic overload

The most common components of food that could cause damage are proteins found in grains, acellular carbohydrates, sugars, genetically modified foods, and conventional dairy products. These foods can cause damage in two ways: they might cause tears in the gut lining that allow bad stuff to leak into the bloodstream, and they might change the makeup of the gut bacteria allowing bad bacteria to overgrow the good bacteria, thereby causing tears in the lining of the gut.

An increase in unhealthy bacteria actually creates toxins called *exotoxins* and *endotoxins* that damage and tear holes in the intestinal wall. Endotoxins from unhealthy gram-negative bacteria are called *lipopolysaccharides*, which are highly inflammatory and toxic to the body.

Other factors that cause leaky gut are chronic stress and external toxic substances.

Stress weakens your immune system over time, which cripples your ability to fight off foreign invaders such as bad bacteria and viruses, leading to inflammation and leaky gut.

External toxic substances are all around us. We come into contact with over 80,000 chemicals (many potentially toxic) every single year. Our body is designed to eliminate most of them. But, it can be overwhelmed by large amounts of toxic substances that the body struggles to eliminate.

Think about a sink that is filling with water. The water flows in but it also flows out through the open drain at the bottom of the sink. If the drain were partially clogged or if the water starts flowing much faster than it can drain out, the sink will overflow, with water ending up everywhere.

In our systems, if toxic substances build up faster than they can be eliminated biologically, they will overflow into areas of the body that never should have been exposed to these toxic substances in the first place. The results are damage to the system. Some of the toxic substances that are most troublesome might surprise you. They include pesticides, household and commercial chemicals, antibiotics, and even some medications such as NSAIDs (non-steroidal anti-inflammatory drugs).

The way to heal a leaky gut is to remove the foods and factors that damage the gut, add nutrient-dense foods in your meals, and support your immune system and overall health with efficient exercise, restorative sleep, and methods to reduce chronic stress.

In summary
- The gut has nerve tissue and chemicals that function like a second brain. Our gut influences how our body feels, and our brain influences how our gut feels.
- We are more bacterial cells than human cells. These bacteria play a critical role in our health, and they must be kept in healthy balance.
- About 70% of the body's immune system resides in the gut.

- If we eat unhealthy foods, we can change the predominantly good bacteria in our gut to predominantly bad bacteria. These bad bacteria--as well as harmful foods, stress, and toxic substances--can damage our gut lining, allowing unwanted substances to leak into our bloodstream. All this can cause a myriad of chronic diseases--not the least of which begins with the gums!

PART II
LIFESTYLE REPAIR

15. Prologue to My Lifestyle-Repair Plan

Statistically, we are living longer in the United States today than ever before, but we are developing chronic diseases that significantly interfere with the quality of our golden years. Some of us are in distress and pain for decades before succumbing to these chronic diseases. This is not the way the human body was designed or evolved to be. We were not born deficient in prescription drugs. We were not born to have to go to the physician every year to stay healthy or to see a dentist twice a year to prevent and treat gum disease and cavities. We were not born to require supplements of vitamins, minerals, and other nutrients for our bodies to function properly.

We were born to be healthy. We were born to retain our adult teeth throughout our lives until we die. We were born to move and jump and run and exert our bodies. We also were born to have pleasure and relax in tune with nature.

Imagine this: You're sitting on your four-legged dining room chair. Notice how you feel: stable and comfortable. But what would happen if one leg suddenly gave out? You'd topple over. How about two legs? Three Legs? You need all four legs of that chair in order to give you the support you need.

Well, your healthy, productive body needs stability too. And, your mouth is just an extension of your functioning body. Your mouth is not an island unto itself; it is intricately and intimately connected to everything that happens to each cell in your body.

Just as there are four legs to a dining room chair, there are four pillars to a healthy "you". Chronic disease occurs when one or more of these pillars are broken. The four pillars are:

- Nutrient-dense real foods
- Restorative sleep
- Efficient exercise
- Stress reduction

Here's a brief description of these four pillars:

- *Nutrient-dense real foods* provide the energy sources that every cell in your body needs to do its thing. These foods consist of wild-caught and free-range animal products from nose to tail along with their wonderful fats. They also include all veggies, some densely colored fruits, plus nuts and seeds in moderation. These foods support your good gut bacteria, critical for good health.

- *Restorative sleep* allows important systems of your body to replenish themselves. Your body needs at least seven to eight hours of sleep every night, ideally in a quiet, cool, dark space. Your body can't function properly if you try to catch up on sleep over the weekend. That's not how it works.

- *Efficient exercise* helps maintain and build your body with the least amount of effort for the maximum effect. A science-based, practical routine could include (first) a ten-to-twenty-minute workout of high-intensity sprinting once every week, plus (second) a ten-to-twenty-minute workout of strength-training exercises twice a week, including squats, pushups, pull-ups, and planks. Also, science has shown that non-exercise movement throughout the day may be as important as efficient exercise. Standing as much as possible and sitting as *little* as possible should become routine. Simple walking is good movement, and a realistic goal to strive for each day should be 10,000 steps, which translates to about 5 miles of walking. A good tool to record how many steps you take every day is a pedometer. My favorite is made by Omron®.

- *Stress reduction* includes the removal of toxic substances from internal and external sources, along with the removal of psychological stresses. Stresses from *any* source are toxic to all cells and eventually to all organs. As these stressors build up in the body to overload the system, clinical manifestations can appear like the proverbial straw that broke the camel's back. These manifestations of toxic overload may be expressed differently for each individual.

Remember: Your body was designed to be a finely tuned machine. These four pillars of health assist every cell in your body to perform as it was meant to perform, resulting in longevity and, most importantly, quality of life. In the next chapter, we'll discuss your very own Lifestyle-Repair Plan, a guide for you to help get your life back on track. This practical program will address all four pillars of health. But first, I have some research to share with you, followed by a few revealing patient stories I think you'll want to hear.

16. Anti-Inflammatory, Nutrient-Dense Diet and Health

There is controversy about the health benefits of a primal or Paleolithic-type diet. Why? There has not been an abundance of peer-reviewed research published. Long-term results, which have proved all the anecdotal health benefits that have been described, need to be reported. Now, new long-term research on humans is being presented in peer-reviewed papers that show profound health benefits from a Paleo-type diet. Also, comparisons of the Paleo-type diet [89] with the Mediterranean diet [90] or with the Diabetes diet[91] have been shown to be superior for the Paleo-type diet.

In support of Paleo-type diets, there are cultures around the world today that are hunter-gatherers or primal societies that demonstrate significant health compared to most civilized societies. In contrast, there are some specific cultures that eat relatively unhealthy foods and who demonstrate documented poor health.

Our primal ancestors did not eat the same foods that we eat. Today's hunter-gatherer or primal societies don't eat the same foods that we eat. Yet, their common thread is that none of their foods consisted of acellular carbohydrates, processed foods, or unhealthy fats. Accordingly, their bodies were and *are* strong, and their overall health is impressive compared to the average U.S. citizen today.

I recently reviewed eight human research articles that begin to bring home the evidence, which I discuss below. Following these human studies, I discuss various societies in the world whose health and diet have been researched and published for the scientific and medical communities. And will *you* be surprised!

Let's look at some facts obtained from peer-reviewed literature, and then you can draw your own conclusions.

Current human research and health

For many years the idea of a Paleo-type diet was observed and anecdotally documented, but well-designed research was lacking. Naysayers said there just wasn't enough concrete evidence to support the claims of those professing a Paleo-type Diet. There was research on animal models, but human studies were lacking. Now, here are the results of the human studies:

Lindeberg, et al in 2007[92] studied 29 men with heart disease and elevated blood sugars. Fourteen men were on a Paleo-type diet and fifteen were on a Mediterranean diet. Both groups could eat as much as they wanted until they were satisfied. After twelve weeks, the Paleo-type group had better control of their blood glucose, which actually returned to normal by the end of the study. Both groups lost weight and inches around their waist, but the Paleo-type group lost more weight and significantly lost more inches around their waists. Interestingly, the Paleo-type group ended up eating significantly fewer calories per day without intentionally restricting calories or portions because their Paleo-type diet was more satiating. They ate more protein and fewer carbohydrates *by choice!*

Osterdahl, et al in 2008[93] looked at fourteen healthy medical students over the course of three weeks. They were instructed to eat a Paleo-type diet. The students' body weight dropped an average of five pounds; their average waist circumference decreased slightly more than half an inch, and their systolic blood pressure dropped an average of three mmHg.

Jonsson, et al in 2009[94] studied thirteen individuals with type 2 diabetes. They were divided into two groups and were placed on either a Paleo-type diet or a typical Diabetes diet in a crossover study. They were on each diet for three months at a time. On the Paleo-type diet, the participants lost 6.6 pounds more weight and lost 1.6 inches more off of their waistlines, compared to the Diabetes diet. In addition:

- HbA1c (a marker for three-month blood sugar levels) decreased by 0.4% more on the Paleo-type diet.

- HDL increased by 3 mg/dL on the Paleo-type diet compared to the Diabetes diet.
- Triglycerides decreased by 35 mg/dL on the Paleo-type diet compared to the Diabetes diet.

Jonsson, et al in 2010[95] studied twenty-nine men with ischemi heart disease who had impaired glucose tolerance or Type 2 diabetes. They were divided into two groups, which were not restricted in how much they could eat: fourteen men were to eat a Paleo-type diet and fifteen, a Mediterranean diet. Each participant recorded his subjective rating of satiety. Those in the Paleolithic group were more satiated per-calorie-consumed compared to those in the Mediterranean group. Leptin decreased by 31% in the Paleolithic group and by 18% in the Mediterranean group. There was a significantly strong correlation in changes in leptin and changes in weight and waist circumference in the Paleolithic group but not in the Mediterranean group.

Frassetto, et al in 2009[96] studied nine healthy individuals. They ate a Paleo-type diet for ten days. In the study, calories were controlled so that the group wouldn't lose weight. Their health results were as follows:

- Total Cholesterol was down 16%.
- LDL Cholesterol was down 22%.
- Triglycerides were down 35%.
- Insulin levels were down 39%.
- Diastolic Blood Pressure was down 3.4 mmHg.

Ryberg, et al in 2013[97] studied ten healthy women who ate a modified Paleo-type diet for five weeks. They lost an average of 9.9 pounds and lost an average of 3.1 inches from around their waists. They also lost an average of 49% of their liver fat. Other health markers were significantly improved:

Mellberg, et al in 2014[98] reported on a two-year study of seventy obese postmenopausal women. This has been the longest study to date where the subjects could eat as much as they wanted.

In this study, the Paleo-type diet was superior to a low fat, high carbohydrate diet for weight loss at six, twelve, and eighteen months and for body fat and waist circumference at six months. The Paleo-type diet caused greater improvements in blood triglycerides after two years than the low fat, high carbohydrate diet. At the conclusion of the two-year study, individuals had increased their dietary protein, reduced their dietary carbohydrates, increased their monounsaturated fats and omega 3-fatty acids, and reduced their omega-6 fatty acids. All these changes have positive health effects on metabolic syndrome diseases, cancer, and autoimmunity.

Boers, et al in 2014[99] selected thirty-four subjects with at least two characteristics of the metabolic syndrome. [100] They were divided into two groups: eighteen ate a Paleo-type diet, and fourteen ate a Dutch Healthy Reference diet[101] for two weeks. Bodyweight was to remain stable as best as possible. The individuals on the Paleo-type diet had the following improvements over those on the Dutch Healthy Reference diet:

- Decreased blood pressure
- Decreased total cholesterol
- Decreased triglycerides
- Increased HDL

Also, the number of characteristics of the metabolic syndrome decreased for those on the Paleo-type diet.

Conclusions from human studies

What does this all mean? These were human studies. Weight decreased; inches around the waist decreased; health markers in the blood improved; blood pressure improved. All markers improved to some extent for subjects who were on a Paleo-type diet. When other diets were compared to the Paleo-type diet, the results for the Paleo-type diet were at least as good as or better than the other diets. Also, those who were on the Paleo-type diet were more satiated per-calorie-consumed than those on other diets. These macro results could only occur if there was improvement on a cellular level first.

Specific cultures and health

A lot can be learned from various cultures regarding the way they eat and their overall health. Many studies have been published describing the foods of various societies around the world, but I have selected eight to summarize. The first is a literature review relating the transition of hunter-gathers to farmers from the recent archeological findings in the Fertile Crescent dating back 10 to 12 thousand years. The next four cultures have consumed foods that were available in their immediate environment, and they have not been exposed to any acellular carbohydrates, processed foods, or unhealthy oils. Their overall health, as you will read, is excellent. The following two societies have been exposed to various amounts of "Westernized" foods. Their health status has been significantly compromised. The last but most recent study compared eye health between a hunter-gatherer society and a neighboring society of farmers in the Amazon.

It is important to remember that most disease begins on a cellular level and transforms into full-blown chronic diseases over time. Specific manifestations of disease are dependent on the individual and his or her weakest biological links. In similar fashion, health also begins on a cellular level. Provide the cells of your body with the nourishment they require, and your overall health benefits.

Gobleki Tepe region of the Fertile Crescent 10,000 years ago[102]. Hugh Freeman reviewed the literature on the emergence of celiac disease (which is a chronic, gluten-based disease primarily affecting the small intestinal mucosa) and published his paper in 2015. Generally the symptoms of celiac disease are diarrhea and weight loss. However, gluten reactions frequently may manifest with few or no intestinal symptoms. Freeman's research of the recent archeological data mainly from the Gobleki Tepe region, indicated that celiac disease probably emerged as humans transitioned from hunter-gatherer groups to societies dependent on agriculture to maintain a stable food supply.

Kitava in the 1990s[103]. Their diet consists of 65% carbohydrates with high fiber and 17% saturated fat. Their food consists mainly of root vegetables, fruit, with some fish and meat, and a large quantity of coconuts. They report no obesity, no strokes, no diabetes, and no heart disease. They experience no increase in blood pressure in middle age.

Machiguenga in 1982.[104]: Their diet mainly consists of high carbohydrates and high fiber. Their foods consists of root vegetables, fruits and nuts, small amounts of meat, and fish. They have no obesity, and they have healthy teeth and gums as well as good overall health.

Masai in 1971[105]. Their diet consists of 66% fat. They eat large amounts of cow's milk and blood, and meat. They are lean and rarely have atherosclerosis when observed at autopsy.

!Kung in 1972[106]. Their diet is 60% fat and 25% protein. Most of their foods are nuts, fruits, roots, leaves, and some meat. They are lean and have no increase in blood pressure through middle age.

Mexican Pima Indians in 2006[107]. Their diet consists of 62% carbohydrates with high fiber and 25% fat. Their foods are high in beans, wheat-flour tortillas, corn tortillas, and potatoes. The incidence of obesity is 7% in males and 20% in females. The overall incidence of diabetes is 7%.

Arizona Pima Indians in 1996-2006[108]. Their diet consists of 49% carbohydrates, 15% protein, and 34% fat. Their foods are refined Western foods such as processed meats, white bread, flour tortillas, fried or baked dough, cereals, canned foods, fruit juices. The obesity rate was 64% in males and 75% in females. The rate of diabetes is greater than 30%. While Arizona's Pima Indians currently have the highest rates of diabetes and obesity in the United States, that wasn't always the case. They were lean until around 1890 when American settlers upstream overtook their water supply. The United States government began subsidizing the tribe's food, much of it containing sugar and white flour. Then, obesity and diabetes rates soared.

Amazonian Kawymeno Waorani and the Kichwa in 2015[109]. Myopia is a condition of decreased visual acuity of the eye where distant objects and images are out of focus, but close-up objects are in focus. This condition is pervasive in modern populations but absent in hunter-gatherer societies today. To study this phenomenon, London and Beezhold compared food systems and visual acuity in a population of hunter-gatherers of the Amazonian Kawymeno Waorani and in the neighboring farmer population of the Kichwa. The hunter-gatherer society consumed significantly more plants (eighty as opposed to four) thereby eating a significantly larger variety and quantity of phytochemicals than did the farming population. Visual acuity was inversely related to age only in the farming group. The hunter-gatherers maintained high visual acuity throughout life, while the visual acuity declined with age in the farming group. The researchers concluded that the intake of a wider variety of plant foods supplying necessary phytochemicals for eye health might help maintain visual acuity and prevent degenerative eye conditions, as humans get older.

Conclusions from specific cultures

In each of these peer-reviewed articles, those cultures that maintained diets of basic hunter-gatherers and primal societies, even though their diets varied in their macronutrient composition, lived relatively healthy lives. Those who changed their diets to include a range of processed foods began to develop various chronic diseases, and their overall health suffered.

Summary

While controversy exists, the research that I have reported throughout this book and in the peer-reviewed literature from this chapter supports a significantly healthier body when it is fed foods of the land and when it is *not* fed foods consisting of acellular carbohydrates, processed foods, and unhealthy fats. Disease starts at the cellular level and can manifest itself as many named diseases, depending on the individual's genetic makeup and other environmental stimuli.

17. Unhealthy Foods Lead to an Unhealthy Body

Unhealthy food choices such as acellular carbohydrates, processed foods, and unhealthy fats have combined over the centuries with a sedentary lifestyle to create a clustering array of symptoms that has become known as the metabolic syndrome.[110] This syndrome is rampant around the world today, and it increases the risk of type-2 diabetes[111,112] and cardiovascular disease.[113]

Metabolic Syndrome is the name for a group of risk factors that raises your risk for heart disease and other health problems.

The five conditions described below are metabolic risk factors. You can have any one of these factors, but they tend most often to occur together. Usually, you must have at least three metabolic risk factors to be diagnosed with metabolic syndrome.

- *A large waistline.* Excess fat in the stomach area is a greater risk factor for heart disease than excess fat in other parts of the body, such as on the hips. Unhealthy carbohydrates play a significant role in forming this waistline, or belly, fat. To see whether or not you fall into this risk category, check out the description below for Waist to Hip Ratio.
- *A high triglyceride level.* Triglycerides are a type of fat found in the blood, and they are elevated predominantly from consuming excess and unhealthy carbohydrates. ("Normal" is <150 mg/dL)
- *A low HDL cholesterol level.* HDL, sometimes is called the "good" cholesterol, helps remove cholesterol from your arteries. A low HDL cholesterol level raises your risk for heart disease. (A level greater than 40-60 mg/dL is desirable--see more below.)
- *High blood pressure.* Blood pressure is the force of the blood pushing against the walls of your arteries as your heart pumps it through the arteries. If this pressure rises and remains high over time, it can damage your heart and lead to plaque buildup and other health problems. (See Table below for BP values.)

- *High fasting blood sugar.* Mildly high blood sugar, which is directly related to the amount and types of carbohydrates you consume, may be an early sign of diabetes. ("Normal" is <100 mg/dL.)

The insulin factor

Insulin is critical for your body to function properly. Insulin resistance occurs when your body's cells don't respond to normal insulin levels, which transports sugar from the bloodstream into muscle and other tissues. As a result, your pancreas begins to produce more insulin to try to force your cells to respond, resulting in excess sugar in your bloodstream. Insulin resistance and chronic low-grade inflammation are increased when you make unhealthy food choices. Bad carbohydrates decrease the ability of your cells and insulin to function properly, actually *increasing* insulin resistance. These unhealthy carbohydrates also damage the gut lining and increase unhealthy forms of bacteria in the gut. Once the gut lining becomes damaged, leaking undigested and harmful food into the bloodstream, chronic inflammation and immune reactions occur. All this leads to metabolic syndrome.[114]

The human studies I described in the previous Chapter have shown that a Paleo-type diet can actually *decrease* these risk factors leading to the Metabolic Syndrome. These diets may be optimal for prevention and treatment of metabolic disorders associated with obesity, type-2 diabetes, cardiovascular disease, and insulin resistance.[115,116,117,118,119,120,121,122]

Some of these studies showed that Paleo-type diets may effectively lower bodyweight, waist circumference and BP,[123] lower serum lipids,[124] and improve insulin response in healthy individuals within less than three weeks.[125] One study[126] demonstrated that the Paleo-type diet lowered most of the metabolic syndrome risk factors in patients with metabolic syndrome in just two weeks while another relatively "healthy" diet did not.

Waist-to-hip ratio measurements

Your waist-to-hip ratio is important because your waist and hip circumferences are important measurements to help determine if you have an increased amount of fat around your belly, indicating an increased health risk. Here's the best way to measure your waist circumference:

- Use a tape measure that has centimeter markings, and place it around your bare stomach at the most-narrow circumference, usually at your belly button or above.
- Look in the mirror to see if the tape measure is parallel to the floor. If you slant the tape, you'll get a false reading. The tape should be snug to your body, but don't compress the skin. Don't hold your stomach in. You want to breath out and relax your stomach.
- Write down your waist circumference in centimeters. Use *centimeters* because they are easier to read and to calculate the ratio.

Your hip circumference

Here's the best way to measure your hip circumference:

- Look in the mirror to determine the widest part of your bare hips.
- Place the tape measure around the widest part. Make sure the tape measure is parallel to the floor. Write down the circumference in centimeters.

Calculate your waist-to-hip ratio

This ratio compares the size of your waist to the size of your hips. The smaller your waist is in comparison to your hips, the lower your risk for heart disease. Even if you're overweight, this ratio is an important measurement.

Calculation:

- Divide your waist circumference in centimeters by your hip circumference in centimeters to determine the Ratio.

- The following table will help you determine your potential health risk.

Waist-to-Hip Ratio and Health Risk		
Male	Female	Risk
0.95 or below	0.80 or below	Low
0.96–1.0	0.81–0.85	Moderate
1.0+	0.85+	High

Triglycerides ÷ HDL Ratio Heart Disease Indicator

It appears common for people with high triglycerides to have low HDL's. In adults, the triglyceride/HDL ratio should be below 2 (divide your level of triglycerides by your level of HDL).

What the triglyceride/HDL ratio means:

- 2 or less is considered ideal
- 4 is high
- 6 is dangerously high

Since HDL (high density lipoprotein) is protective against heart disease, the lower the triglyceride/HDL ratio, the better. In other words, the lower your triglycerides, or the higher your HDL, the smaller this ratio becomes.

The triglyceride/HDL ratio is one of the more important predictors of heart disease. [127] A Harvard-led study author reported:

"High triglycerides alone increased the risk of heart attack nearly three-fold. And people with the highest ratio of triglycerides to HDL had 16 times the risk of heart attack as those with the lowest ratio of triglycerides to HDL in the study of 340 heart attack patients and 340 of their healthy, same age counterparts. The ratio of triglycerides to HDL was the strongest predictor of a heart attack, even more accurate than the LDL/HDL ratio."

Resting Blood Pressure for Adults From "Normal" to "Stage 2 High Blood Pressure" (measured in millimeters of mercury, or mmHg)			
Category	Systolic (top number)		Diastolic (bottom number)
Normal	Less than 120	*And*	Less than 80
Prehypertension	120–139	*Or*	80–89
High blood pressure			
Stage 1	140–159	*Or*	90–99
Stage 2	160 or higher	*Or*	100 or higher

18. What My Patients Are Saying

When I first decided to include this chapter in the book, I wondered if I would have enough serious questions, comments, and concerns from the people who come to my office for a professional visit. I needn't have bothered. Here are just a few of the things they're saying, and some of my comments regarding their concerns.

My gums became suddenly swollen

I first examined a 45-year old woman named Christine in 2010. Her gums were not bleeding or swollen, but her complaint was that her gums were receding around her teeth, which was exposing her root surfaces. She was concerned, even though she didn't have any tooth sensitivity.

After examining her, I discovered she was a severe "grinder." The rocking forces on her teeth that she created by grinding mainly when she was sleeping were causing damage to the super-thin bone on the cheek surfaces of her teeth that were located in the back of her mouth. When this thin bone was destroyed from the tooth rocking against it, the gum tissues around the teeth in question actually shrank and receded. I suggested the following treatment: (1) Allow me to smooth the chewing surfaces of her teeth so they would come together more evenly, and (2) Let me construct a "bite guard" made from molds of her teeth--something she would wear whenever she was sleeping so that any grinding forces would let her teeth glide on the bite guard surface and prevent her from rocking her teeth in her jawbone. She appeared to understand why I thought that her gums were receding, and she told me that she would think about it.

She did not accept my treatment, and I did not see her again until 2014, nearly four years later. A year or so after I had seen her in 2010, she had suffered a significant crisis: her husband died suddenly. When she finally returned to see me, she had a different complaint. She explained to me that she had suddenly developed severe swelling and redness in her gum tissues throughout her mouth. She said she was taking several new antidepressant medications, and that she constantly tired. I suggested that the new medications could have caused her new symptoms. I also suggested there could be underlying medical problems as well as dietary problems that could have caused the new symptoms so suddenly. I wanted her to see her medical doctor for a complete exam to rule out any other possible systemic problems.

She postponed her appointment with her medical doctor. Three weeks later, she informed my office that she was feeling so weak that she had to go to the emergency room. She was diagnosed with leukemia.

I tell this story because most of the time gum inflammation and gum swelling are the results of bacterial infection and improper diet. However, rarely there may be an underlying serious disease causing these problems. All patients need to have a thorough medical examination to rule out the unusual when they're experiencing unusually strange or severe symptoms.

My gums are bleeding and sore

About a year ago, I was asked to evaluate a patient who had bleeding gums, which were not responding to daily, good oral hygiene and had not responded to a deep cleaning by the hygienist in his dentist's office.

This 71-year old gentleman named Gene had ongoing gum issues that were documented for more than three years. More likely than not, they had begun decades before. When I spoke to him, he did not complain of pain all the time, but he explained that his gums would bleed when he brushed his teeth and were a little sore. He wanted a quick fix like an antibiotic.

I told him we first needed to rule out infections and any blood diseases including anything serious, such as cancer. As I questioned him, he told me that he had bouts of diarrhea and bloating. He also complained of acid reflux disease for which his medical doctor put him on an acid-reducing prescription. When I questioned him about his eating habits, he told me he had a healthy bowl of oatmeal every morning and usually some pasta dish with dinner. I suggested that some of his gum problem could be coming from the grains that he was eating.

He immediately dismissed my idea. He said he had been eating that way his entire life; therefore, that obviously could not be at the cause of his gum sores. He left my office to seek other opinions.

Several months later, I saw him again. He had seen an oral surgeon and then his own medical doctor who put him on anti-inflammatory prescription drugs. The meds failed to cure the bleeding, and he finally allowed me to make some suggestions.

I had him fill out a three-day food journal listing everything he ate. He also had to write down the frequency of his bowel movements and any exercise he participated in during these three days. When I reviewed his journal with him, we discovered he was eating some type of grain product with every meal as well as at every snack. We also saw how few green vegetables he was consuming. Most of his drinks were laden with sugar.

I had him promise to do an experiment for thirty days. Since he had been suffering with bleeding and sore gums for several years, it didn't seem all that great a hardship. Here's the plan I put him on.

- Eliminate all grains. I described the foods that had grains and grain products that had to be eliminated. I also gave him a list of foods that could be substituted for these grains and snacks. I even included some of my favorite recipes.
- Eliminate all sugary drinks. I recommended various drinks including regular water that he should be drinking.
- Take a nutrient-dense supplement. This consisted of *fermented* cod liver oil capsules as well as organic kelp powder capsules every day. I gave him resources online where he could purchase them.
- Use coconut oil as a mouthwash. He was to place half a teaspoon of the oil in his mouth and swish. After a few

minutes, he was to spit it out into a napkin and not into the sink where the oil might clog the drain. After that, he would rinse with warm water. He was to do that several times a day if possible.

At the end of the thirty-day period, we agreed to meet again and evaluate his progress. When the time came, he was amazed to admit his bleeding gums were significantly better than before, not yet healed, but on their way. My further discussions with him were to include improving the bacteria in his gut and continuing to modify his diet to remove all offending items and replace what needed to be there. If necessary at a later date, I told him I would suggest some functional medicine testing to delve into specific cellular problems. His progress has been remarkable.

I thought I could cheat with grains

This story drives home the point that what goes into (or *doesn't* go into) our guts could be severely damaging to other parts of our body, starting with our gum tissues. A former patient of one of my colleagues related these comments to me.

For the last two years, I have been on a gluten-free diet because of problems I had with irritable bowel syndrome (IBS). I have been tested for celiac disease, but there was no definitive diagnosis. But, once I became gluten-free, my IBS seemed to get better. So, I thought that after two years I could start to eat some of the baked goods that I used to love. What a mistake!

While at one of my favorite restaurants, I had a dinner roll with my meal. The next day, not having any problems, I bought a bagel for breakfast at my favorite coffee shop. Then, here and there, some more cheating.

About a month later, my gums were starting to get very sore and would bleed easily. Bleeding gums have always been a problem for me on and off. So, I went to my dentist to check it out. He seemed concerned and referred me to an oral surgeon to have a biopsy. The results came back as Mucous Membrane Pemphigoid (MMP).

I realized that these problems only became obvious after I started eating bread products about a month ago. Could the gum problem and the grains be related?

Mucous Membrane Pemphigoid (MMP) is an autoimmune disease of the mucous membranes, and it can affect any part of the body that has mucous membranes, such as the eyes, mouth, nose, digestive tract, and anus. The medical community has not defined an exact cause of this disease. Treatment by medical professionals usually involves medicines to control inflammation and to reduce pain. However, as with most autoimmune diseases, permeability of the gut (leaky gut) could be the ultimate source of this disease.

The manifestation of a gut-lining problem caused by grain consumption could make itself known with differing diagnoses and symptoms. The manifestations could show themselves as bleeding gums, a skin lesion such as psoriasis, or even a glandular problem such as hypothyroidism. You may develop joint soreness, headaches, or general fatigue. In the patient's story above, a leaky gut could have caused or exacerbated MMP. Your weakest cells or your most vulnerable areas would most likely be the affected parts. Most importantly, you don't have to experience gut discomfort or pain to have a gut-lining problem that causes chronic or autoimmune diseases in other locations of your body.

The bottom line is to heal the gut first, after which a healing process can begin for other symptoms. Be aware that grain products that have damaged the gut lining in the past will continue to wreak havoc in the body in the future. If you have eliminated grain products but reintroduced them, even in minute quantities, that could set off cascading effects throughout your body. It is not only critical to eat the right foods, but also critical to avoid the bad foods *forever*. For this patient, completely refraining from grain products as well as other foods that may have cross-reactivity turned out prudent.

My life is so stressful!

The following pictures may be disturbing to some readers because they may look unnatural. The photography was done with the lips pulled back to show the teeth and gums for better viewing.

In this mouth of a thirty-something woman, Doris visited her periodontist, Dr. J. Daulton Keith, complaining of sore, swollen, bleeding gums. There were no obvious causes for this problem; she had very little dental plaque around her gum tissues and did not have any obvious nutritional deficiencies. Dr. Keith referred her to her medical doctor to check for possible systemic diseases that could be sources of her mouth problem.

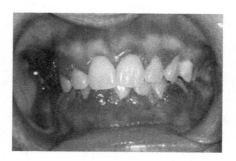

Her MD ran various blood tests and determined that there were no medical conditions he could find that were the cause of her unhealthy gum tissues. After she returned to Dr. Keith's office, she broke down crying and described the emotional and sexual abuse she had to endure from her employer. Dr. Keith convinced her to make a life change. She was fortunate and able to secure excellent employment with a different company in another state, to quit her job with her abusive employer, and to relocate within a short period of time.

Four months later, she returned to Dr. Keith's office. From the time she originally was seen by Dr. Keith to the time she returned after her move, she did not receive any medical or dental treatment for her mouth lesions. Her only treatment was the removal of her emotional stress.

Here is the picture of her mouth after she returned to the periodontal office. All of the gum lesions were gone--no soreness; no bleeding; no lesions. Her original mouth condition had been caused by nothing more than severe emotional stress overloading her body's ability to cope. Her cure was the direct result of totally eliminating this stress from her life.

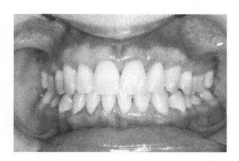

Unfortunately, most people who experience emotional stress from whatever sources are unable to reduce that stress completely. Fortunately for Doris, she was!

By now, you're beginning to see how many variables can go into causing various gum diseases. Hopefully, you're also beginning to see that, for every problem, there *is* a solution. Let's take a look at my *Lifestyle-Repair Plan* that includes diet and lifestyle principles that can affect your good health, and your life, forever.

19. The Lifestyle-Repair Plan

My *Plan* is made up of three major sections, which are further subdivided. The names of each section form the acronym, GUM, which as a periodontist pleases me to no end. The acronym is short for three little words: Give, Undo, and Master.

- *GIVE* yourself nutrient-dense nourishment. By providing your body with the right, healthy nutrition, you're providing it with the tools necessary to grow and remain healthy.
- *UNDO* the damage. This refers to removing bad food choices, toxic substances, irritants, and unhealthy stresses from your life.
- *MASTER* the methods of maintenance details a lifestyle incorporating good oral hygiene, effective exercise, non-exercise movement, restorative sleep, and stress reduction.

Think about getting your entire family onboard with The Lifestyle-Repair Plan. The more members of your immediate household participate, the easier it will be to make permanent lifestyle changes for everyone! Let's take a closer look.

G - GIVE yourself nutrient-dense nourishment!

The foods that were essential for our primal ancestors, the ones that maintained healthy bacteria in their bodies and provided the fuel for cells to function at their peak levels, are still the foods our present-day bodies need to thrive. These nutrient-dense foods include animals from head to tail that have been pastured in their natural settings and able to eat their natural diets. Also included are vegetables, fruits, nuts, and seeds. The best choices are locally grown and raised without chemicals, antibiotics, hormones, or pesticides.

Nutrient density means how many nutrients are in a food, given the number of calories it contains. It's a simple way to connect nutrients with calories. In other words, nutrient dense foods give you the "biggest bang for the buck." You get lots of nutrients, and it doesn't cost you much in terms of calories.

Nutrients can be divided into macronutrients and micronutrients:

- Macronutrients are energy-providing chemical substances consumed in large quantities. The three macronutrients in nutrition are carbohydrates, fats and oils, and proteins.
- Micronutrients are necessary only in small amounts but are critical for good health. They are commonly referred to as vitamins and minerals and also include trace elements.

Our primal ancestors had a diverse diet based on where they lived. Some diets were high in healthy carbs; some were high in healthy fats; some were high in healthy protein sources. Yet, everyone survived and thrived. Hunter-gatherer and primal societies today also have diversity in their food choices. However, the things that none of our primal ancestors or modern-day hunter-gatherers ate were dense, acellular carbohydrates or processed foods. They also were not exposed to an abundance of toxic substances that overstressed their bodies. It is probably more important to *avoid specific things* (which I describe in *U: UNDO the Damage!*) and then *to create good habits* (*M: MASTER Methods of Maintenance!*) than it is to eat only specific healthy foods. All that said, anti-inflammatory, nutrient-dense foods contain all the nutrients our bodies need.

I divided this chapter into nutrient-dense food categories to include in your daily way of eating. I have not suggested specific *foods* you must eat but rather included specific *categories* of foods. Your tastes will dictate what you eat, but I have included in the Appendix of this book some of my favorite recipes that I prepare regularly. Remember, it is most important to avoid the harmful "foods" I describe in the next Chapter.

Here are some interesting facts about all plants, which includes vegetables, fruits, nuts, and seeds.

- Plants manufacture phytonutrients inside their cells. These phytonutrients are like the immune cells in our bodies, and there are more than 25,000 different phytonutrients found in plants[128], with more being discovered all the time. These nutrients help the plants to fight infections and maintain their health. Our body benefits significantly from many of these phytonutrients when we eat plants. They have health-promoting properties including antioxidant, anti-inflammatory, and other biological activities. The deep colors in plants represent the intensity of the phytonutrients available to us.

- If plants are exposed to many insults from their environment, they develop more intense phytonutrients for self-protection. If plants are not exposed to these insults, they develop fewer phytonutrients. When plants are sprayed with insecticides and other chemicals to kill off predators and microbes, these plants not only have a chemical residue that is not healthy for humans, they also produce fewer phytonutrients. Eating organic not only reduces our toxic consumption but also increases the quantity and quality of the phytonutrients in these organically grown plants. Locally grown is better than grown thousands of miles away because locally grown is fresher, and those plants grown many miles away are picked well before their peak ripeness and maximum nutrient benefits for the purposes of not spoiling over long shipping distances.

Before I discuss my suggestions for nutrient-dense food categories, first think about this. Eating nutrient-dense foods will *not* involve counting calories or weighing foods. Our primal ancestors didn't know macronutrients from macaroons. They certainly didn't know anything about grams of protein or Vitamin D levels or the amount of omega-3 fatty acids in their salmon. They knew that, when they were hungry, they ate. They knew that, when they were satisfied, they stopped. They knew that, when they were thirsty, they drank. Their healthy lifestyles balanced their hormones and made them strong. Balanced hormones communicated with their brains to tell them when to stop eating and when to eat again. Primal humans did not have a set time for breakfast, lunch, or dinner. Yet, as I have said before, our primal ancestors hardly ever had gum disease, tooth decay, or chronic diseases.

However, since most of us are deficient in many nutrient-dense foods and are used to eating a relatively unbalanced and compromised diet, here is a way to start thinking about how to eat with healthy food choices:

Every time you eat, either a regular meal or a snack, think of it as "a plate of food." Ideally, the types of food on that "plate" should be balanced as follows:

- At least half the plate should be non-starchy vegetables, cooked or raw, with some additional healthy fat, such as grass-fed butter or olive oil.
- A quarter or less of the plate should be a protein source with all of its healthy fats.
- The last quarter or less should consist of deeply colored fruits and/or nuts and seeds and/or a starchy vegetable along with additional healthy fats, such as butter from grass-fed cattle.

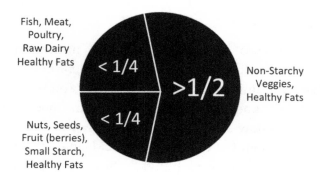

Our body knows what it needs. It also knows to tell you when to stop because you are satiated--not stuffed. The most efficient way to get nourishment is to eat the foods that have the most nutrients as possible from our environment. That means to eat foods that are nutrient-dense.

You will notice that *carbohydrates* are not included as a nutrient-dense food category. The human species has never had a need for a specific amount of *essential carbohydrates* in the diet. It is possible to live a healthy life never consuming much in the way of extra carbohydrates as long as you get adequate dietary protein and fat and eat a variety of vegetables and fruits. Protein and fat were the dominant macronutrients over the majority of 2.5 million years of human evolution. If the body needed additional glucose, the liver was able to create it from fats and proteins (called *gluconeogenesis*). All the carbohydrates necessary for a healthy life could be derived from the cells of vegetables and fruits.

Here are nutrient-dense food categories that have maintained healthy bodies since the day human beings became human beings. It's hardly a fad diet; it's a lifestyle.

Animal protein

Animal foods offer the best forms of healthy protein as well as fat for your body. They provide significant amounts of protein and all types of essential fatty acids, vitamins, and minerals, and they don't stimulate overproduction of insulin. Animal sources will help to reduce excess body fat, build lean muscle, and generally promote peak performance. All primal societies have survived on some type and some amount of animal proteins. There has never been a primal society that restricted animal protein completely.[129]

Animals raised locally that have been pastured or wild caught are the best food choices. Cattle should be grass-fed and grass-finished (which means they have never been fed grains); pork should be pastured and allowed to feed naturally; chickens should be allowed to eat bugs from the ground without being caged and without being fed unnatural foods; fish should be wild caught, not farm-raised. Protein from grass-fed and grass-finished meats, wild caught shellfish and fish (especially small varieties such as sardines, herring, and anchovies), pastured chickens and their eggs, and pastured hogs contain necessary nutrients that need to be included in your diet. I'll share some great recipes with you in the back of the book.

The most important concept you need to understand is this: Conventionally raised animals that have been caged and fed unnatural diets (in conflict with their individual digestive needs) contain harmful products that are destructive to our bodies once we ingest them. Therefore, *don't ingest them!*

Organ meats

Hunter-gatherer societies today often throw away the muscular parts of their kill and eat the organs raw. Why is this? Because, organ meats are the most nutrient-dense parts of the animal. They didn't read this in a book. They happen to know it from thousands of years of their society's healthy life experience. This type of diet supplies two to ten times the recommended daily allowance of vitamins and nutrients.[130,131]

Organ meats can offset the negative effects of excess *methionine* (an amino acid that is abundant in lean meats and eggs). Excess methionine has been shown to increase the incidence of cancer and decrease lifespan in various studies.[132,133] Organ meats provide (among many other nutrients) glycine, B vitamins, choline, and betaine, which have the benefit of balancing out excess methionine in the diet.

Gelatin from organ meats is also beneficial for healing your gut, maintaining healthy skin, protecting your skin, and increasing the quality of your sleep.

Organ meats may be difficult to get used to eating because we are not accustomed to them. However, if you eat oysters and mussels, you are eating their organs along with their meat. If you eat sardines in a can, you are eating some of their organs. You could buy cooked dried whole anchovies from an Asian market, and you would be eating the whole fish, which includes their organs. If you eat bone broth, you are consuming some bone marrow and cartilage, which are organ foods. Oxtail (cow tail) is delicious and provides an abundance of organ-meat benefits. Heart, liver, and kidney--all can be made into delicious and tempting dishes. If necessary, you could disguise organ meats in recipes like I do in my *French Onion Oxtail Slow-Cooker Stew*, *Paleo Four-Meat Chili*, *Slow Cooker Meatloaf Wrapped in Bacon*, and *Slow-Cooker Bone Broth* recipes. These and many more such recipes appear later in the book.

Healthy fats and oils

What's the difference between *fats* and *oils*? Simply this: fats are solid at room temperature and oils are liquid at room temperature. However, the terms are often used interchangeably.

Fats are compounds of carbon, hydrogen, and oxygen atoms that exist in chains varying in length, shapes, and orders. They are required for many bodily functions including energy and cell membrane integrity.

Fats are classified as being saturated, monounsaturated, and polyunsaturated. (There is an unsaturated fat that has a variant structure known as a *trans-fat* that I will discuss at the end of this section.) However, it is important to understand that all naturally occurring fats to some extent contain both saturated and unsaturated elements. The ratios are critical, and the dominant level of saturation is what classifies the category of the fat in question. For example, if a fat's ratio of elements (*saturated* to *monounsaturated* to *polyunsaturated*) is 30:65:5 percent, it would be classified as a monounsaturated fat since the predominant component is 65 percent monounsaturated.

1. Saturated fats are critical for the human body. They make up half of our cell membrane structure, enhance calcium absorption and immune function, and provide cholesterol as well as a rich source of fat-soluble vitamins. These saturated fats have been demonized in the past; they have been considered unhealthy and disease-promoting. Misrepresented research in the past suggested that saturated fats made you fat and also created heart disease.

Actually, unhealthy fats will make you fatter, especially if you are eating dense, acellular carbs (flour, sugar products, and processed foods). A recent systematic review and meta-analysis[134] has disproven the theory that saturated fats are unhealthy. Unfortunately, the theory that saturated fat is unhealthy is still being perpetuated. The fact is that saturated fats from pastured and wild-caught animals and some plants are necessary for many biological functions. If you were eating products from animals that were conventionally raised (that is, fed with unnatural feed and given antibiotics and hormones), then their saturated fats would be unhealthy.

2. Monounsaturated fats are more stable than polyunsaturated fats. It is important to know how much monounsaturated fat is in the makeup of a particular oil. Look at these examples of olive oil compared to corn oil:

   o Olive oil contains about 75% monounsaturated fat, 14% saturated fat, and 11% polyunsaturated fat. Olive oil's ratio of omega-6 to omega-3 in the polyunsaturated component is 4:1. Olive oil is considered relatively healthy.

   o Corn oil, on the other hand, contains about 29% monounsaturated fat, 14% saturated fat, and 57% polyunsaturated fat. Corn oil's ratio of omega-6 to omega-3 in the polyunsaturated component is 46:1. Corn oil is considered unhealthy and unstable.

3. Polyunsaturated fatty acids (PUFAs) run the gamut from good to ugly, from fatty fish and nuts to corn and canola oils. They are easily damaged when they are produced commercially, and they tend to go rancid especially when heated during cooking or when exposed to air, light, and moisture. The resulting damage encourages oxidation, a process that creates free radicals. Free radicals make their way through the body damaging everything from cell membranes and DNA/RNA strands to blood vessels. The harm adds up over time in the organs and systems of the

body and can cause significant impact, including premature aging and skin disease, liver damage, immune dysfunction, and even cancer.

Now, I'm going to get technical.

Polyunsaturated fatty acids have more than one double-bonded carbon link that is missing its hydrogen atom. If there were no double-bonded carbon links, the fat would be saturated; if there were only one double-bonded carbon link, it would be a monounsaturated fat. Because polyunsaturated fats have multiple "incomplete" double bonds each missing a hydrogen atom, they are generally chemically unstable and prone to oxidation. This is why some of them are harmful for our body's chemistry.

Polyunsaturated fatty acids are classified into various biologically important subgroups, especially: omega-6 and omega-3 fatty acids. It is important to note that specific PUFAs are essential for our body. The Essential Fatty Acids are those that our body can't produce and must obtain from food. These essential fatty acids can be made into other necessary fatty acids by the liver. The omega-6 fatty acid that is essential is called linoleic acid (LA), and the omega-3 fatty acid that is essential is called alpha linolenic acid (ALA). However, ratios are critical. Too much of omega-6 fatty acids are inflammatory. What keeps the ratio in check is the amount of omega-3 you consume. A healthy ratio of omega-6 to omega-3 is from 1:1 to 3:1. The Standard American Diet averages anywhere from 10-30 parts of omega-6 to 1 part omega-3 (10-30:1). Our primal ancestors likely enjoyed a ratio close to 1:1. It all comes down to a balance of omega-6 to omega-3 fatty acids.

Three important forms of omega-3 fatty acids are: ALA (*alpha linolenic acid*, as in flaxseed oil) as well as EPA and DHA (as in cold-water fatty fish and fish oil). EPA is *eicosapentaenoic acid*, and DHA is *docosahexaenoic acid*. Both are necessary throughout life, and DHA can be synthesized from EPA. ALA, which is an essential fatty acid, can be converted into EPA and DHA but with difficulty. It is best to get EPA and DHA from natural sources of fatty fish (found in salmon, sardines, herring, anchovies, and cod liver and krill oil). Omega-3s aid circulation by naturally thinning the blood, fighting systemic inflammation, supporting brain function and easing symptoms of depression, anxiety and even ADHD.

Hunter-gatherers from primal beings to present-day societies have eaten mostly saturated fats. They got their essential fatty acids from wild caught fish and pastured animals. A few nuts and seeds rounded out their sources for essential fatty acids. Today, we overdose on PUFAs with all the vegetable oils we use (examples: corn, canola, soybean, sunflower, and safflower) as well as artificial butter products, grain-fed animal fat, and other modern processed foods. A limited amount of nuts and seeds is OK. But, avoiding excess PUFAs in general is a good rule of thumb.

Healthy omega-6 fatty acids are found primarily in nuts and seeds, and healthy omega-3 fatty acids are found primarily in fatty fish, algae, flax, and nuts. Also, significant amounts of healthy omega-3s are found in eggs from chickens that are pastured as well as in grass-fed/grass-finished beef.

The best way to combat an excess of omega-6 in the foods you eat is to watch your ratios and to consume more omega-3s.

PUFA summary

These fats are generally chemically unstable. As I stated, there are some naturally occurring polyunsaturated fats that are necessary for our health since they cannot be manufactured by our bodies. They are LA (an omega-6 fatty acid) and ALA (an omega-3 fatty acid). We need to ingest sources of these essential fatty acids as well as EPA and DHA that are fresh. If not fresh, they could be damaging to our bodies because their chemical structures could be breaking down. Omega-6 is more inflammatory, and omega-3 is more anti-inflammatory--but both are essential. The secret is that they should be consumed in the ratio of about 1:1 (Omega-6:Omega-3). If we were consuming an average ratio that significantly favored omega-6 over omega-3, then bad things would begin to happen on a cellular level. Unfortunately, in our

Standard American Diet, the ratio is out of whack at about 10-30:1 (Omega-6:Omega-3).

Following is a sampling of oils and their fat breakdown[135]:

Oil	Sat. Fat	Mono Fat	Poly. Fat	Omega-6: Omega-3
Avocado	12%	74%	14%	13:1
Canola	8%	64%	28%	2:1
Coconut	92%	6%	2%	No Omega-3
Corn	14%	29%	57%	46:1
Cottonseed	27%	19%	54%	258:1
Grapeseed	10%	17%	73%	696:1
Olive	14%	75%	11%	13:1
Red Palm	52%	37%	11%	46:1
Peanut	18%	49%	33%	No Omega-3
Soybean	16%	24%	60%	8:1
Safflower	7%	15%	78%	No Omega-3
Sesame	15%	41%	44%	138:1
Sunflower	10%	60%	30%	781:1
Walnut	10%	24%	66%	5:1

We need to eat all forms of healthy fats, in which many essential micronutrients reside. Healthy fats made up as much as 60% of calories in some of our primal ancestors' diets. Healthy fats are found in avocados, coconut oil, olive oil, wild-caught oily fish such as salmon, organ foods such as liver and brain from pastured animals, butter from grass-fed cows, eggs from pastured chickens, muscle meat from pastured animals, and some nuts and seeds.

Trans fats

To complete a discussion of healthy fats, I need to include *trans fats*. Trans fats are structurally modified unsaturated fats. Generally, they are not found in nature. There is a naturally-occurring trans-fat called *conjugated linoleic acid*--CLA--that is found in grass-fed meat and dairy products. There is also a naturally-occurring trans-fat called *conjugated linolenic acid*--CLnA--which is found in pomegranates[136]. These are healthy fats that should not be confused with commercially manufactured, toxic trans fats.

Commercially manufactured trans fats are not natural and are toxic to our body. These fats go through a process of hydrogenation making them more solid and their products more shelf stable. However, these fats have caused severe damage to our cells by passing through their membranes and disrupting cell metabolism. Avoid anything chemically altered, commercially manufactured, or products that state "hydrogenated" or "partially hydrogenated" on the label.

Non-starchy vegetables

The micronutrients in non-starchy vegetables provide essential building blocks for our individual cells. These vegetables also provide necessary fibers for our gut and gut bacteria. Non-starchy vegetables have a much lower carbohydrate density than starchy vegetables.

Non-starchy vegetables are typically flowering parts of the plant. Examples are lettuce, asparagus, broccoli, cauliflower, cucumber, spinach, mushrooms, onions, peppers, and tomatoes. Starchy vegetables, on the other hand, are high-carbohydrate plant foods and can contribute to weight gain and increased levels of blood glucose. Examples are peas, yams, potatoes, and plantains. On the other hand, though, starchy vegetables can supply healthy fibers for the gut bacteria.

Locally grown organic varieties of non-starchy vegetables are best. Leafy green vegetables are great, but also select as many different and dark colors as you can. Different colors represent various necessary phytonutrients. A great way to "eat" your veggies is to "drink" some of them in a smoothie. I list my favorite smoothie recipes in the Appendix.

Sea vegetables (seaweed)

Sea vegetables have ready access to the abundance of minerals found in the ocean. Seawater and human blood contain many of the same minerals in very similar concentrations, but most of us don't know much about sea veggies.

Sea vegetables (seaweeds) are unique because of their abundance of trace minerals that many of us are lacking. They provide most of the minerals and trace minerals required for the body's physiological functions, and they contain ten to twenty times the minerals of some land plants.[137] Also, their minerals have been shown to be more bioavailable than most other mineral sources.[138]

These unique vegetables provide many health benefits. They have antioxidant and anti-inflammatory properties, inhibit absorption of toxic substances, are a good source of natural iodine, strengthen the immune system, and reduce the risk of cardiac diseases. Examples of edible seaweeds are nori, wakame, kelp, and dulse. You might want to try my seaweed soup recipe in the back of the book.

Fruits

Fruits are generally healthy, but they are high in carbohydrates and should be eaten in moderation. Their level of carbohydrates can be a concern especially if you are trying to lose weight.

Like vegetables, fruits are plants with a wealth of phytonutrients. As with vegetables, organically grown fruits are healthier than non-organically grown fruits, and locally grown is better than fruits that are grown from thousands of miles away.

A good rule of thumb is to eat fruit that is deeply colored throughout the meat of the fruit. The deep color suggests the intensity of the phytonutrients that are available. The best choices are all berries (such as strawberries, blueberries, blackberries, raspberries) as well as citrus.

A special case for pomegranates

The pomegranate is a food that has benefits for those who want to prevent gum disease or who already have gum disease or other serious ailments. A paper that was published in the July-August 2014 issue of the *Journal of Indian Society of Periodontology* summarized sixty-five peer-reviewed articles to come up with some amazing facts and conclusions.[139]

Pomegranates are one of the oldest edible fruits, which have a long history of medicinal value. Many fruits are nature's gift to health, and pomegranates are one of the best. They have various bioactive components, which possess documented medicinal benefits with minimal side effects.[140]

Several studies have shown that elements in pomegranates will reduce gingival bleeding and pocket depths.[141, 142, 143] Rinses containing extracts of pomegranates have been shown to be as antibacterial as *chlorhexidine*.[144,145]

Pomegranates also could be an excellent adjunct to conventional periodontal therapy as an anti-plaque agent due to their antibacterial properties and their ability to prevent the attachment of plaque's biofilm to the tooth surface.[146]

Deep periodontal pockets have been shown to be associated with *Helicobacter pylori* (*H. pylori*) infection--the primary cause of ulcers.[147] Increased levels of *H. pylori* also have been detected in the mouths of patients with periodontitis.[148,149,150] Pomegranates have demonstrated significant antibacterial activity against *H. pylori*.[151]

In addition, pomegranates have demonstrated positive effects on healthy gut bacteria.[152] By increasing healthy gut bacteria, periodontal pathogens are reduced.[153]

But pomegranates are not just for gum disease. They have significant benefits for overall health. Pomegranates have been considered "a pharmacy unto itself"[154] because they possess bactericidal, antifungal, antiviral, and anti-inflammatory properties. While the natural phytochemicals in pomegranates have proven to be good alternatives to many synthetic antimicrobials[155], they may prevent bacteria from becoming antibiotic resistant.[156] They also have been widely used in the treatment of cardiovascular diseases, diabetes, asthma, inflammation, ulcers, mouth lesions, skin lesions, atherosclerosis, hypertension, hyperlipidemia, Alzheimer's disease, obesity, and many more.[157,158,159]

Let's get to the actual fruit.

A ripe pomegranate is about five inches wide with a deep red, leathery skin. The fruit inside contains many seeds separated by white, membranous pericarp. The seeds are enclosed in small, red, jewel-like drops called arils. The material inside the arils is tart and juicy and surrounds the white seeds of the pomegranate fruit. The arils and crunchy white seeds are the only edible portions of the pomegranate. Yummy, tart, and healthy!

Here is how to open the pomegranate and remove the arils.[160] Be careful. The liquid part of the arils will stain everything!

- Cut off its flowery crown and stem base with a sharp knife.
- Score the pomegranate with cuts from the crown area to the base of the fruit as if you are going to break it into quarters. Don't cut too deeply, or you will injure the arils.
- Soak it in cold water in a large bowl. The water will loosen the seeds to make them easier to collect.
- While the pomegranate is under water, gently pull fruit apart into quarters. This also prevents you from dripping the liquid that will stain.
- Run your fingers through each quarter slice to start separating the seeds while still in the water bath.
- Remove the white, fibrous material, which should mostly be floating on the top of the water.
- Use a strainer to gather the arils.
- Air dry for 5 minutes on a paper towel.
- Store the seeds if you don't want to eat them right away. You can lay them flat in a container and refrigerate them for up to three days, or freeze them for up to six months.

I love the whole fruit. I don't suggest taking supplements containing extracts of pomegranates. I don't suggest drinking the juice of pomegranates. I do recommend that you eat pomegranates--the arils and the crunchy seeds. It is always healthier eating a fruit rather than drinking its juice. Juice is loaded with sugars and devoid of many nutrients that juicing discards.

A special case for local, raw honey

Honey! It's sticky, sweet, and yummy. Is it a confection, or is it a powerful medicine?

It's both.

Interestingly, the anecdotal health reports over the centuries are now supported by clinical trials. The peer-reviewed articles I researched were not sensational; they very well may have been understated. Read the facts; then you decide.[161]

It all started a long time ago. Recorded history about honey's medicinal and antimicrobial properties for wound healing goes back about 5000 years. However, the use of honey as a food and as a medicine probably goes back to the beginning of primal societies who discovered this luscious, nutrient-dense food of the bees.

Honey is a supersaturated nectar collected by honeybees from a wide variety of plants. The actual composition of honey depends on the composition of the nectar collected from specific flowers around the world. The highest percentages of components are fructose (about 38%) and glucose (about 31%).

It is surprising that such a sweet, sugar-laden food could offer so many medicinal properties. While these biological processes are still not well understood, honey's benefits have been demonstrated in many recently published, peer-reviewed studies.

In addition to fructose and glucose, there are over 180 substances that have been identified in raw honey. No doubt, many have yet to be discovered. Some of the compounds contained in honey include sugars (other than fructose and glucose), phenolic acids, flavonoids, amino acids, proteins, vitamins, and enzymes, all of which synergistically account for honey's biological effects. The benefits include antimicrobial, anti-inflammatory, anti-allergic, antithrombotic, and vasodilatory actions.[162]

Honey also stimulates wound healing even in wounds that have not responded to other treatments. Some of the unique qualities of honey that may be at work here are its acidic level (pH of 3.2 to 4.5), its activation of the immune system, and its promotion of cell growth.[163]

Eating honey can improve cardiovascular risk. Consuming honey has been shown to increase HDL cholesterol, reduce LDL cholesterol, and reduce triglycerides.[164,165]

Even type 1 and type 2 diabetics have benefited from the inclusion of honey in their diets.[166,167]

With all the sugar, one would think that honey would cause gum disease and dental decay. But, the facts are just the opposite.

In this randomized, control study, patients were given one of three different sweeteners to eat--honey, sorbitol, or sucrose. The results were surprising. Eating honey actually *decreased* the bacteria that caused gum disease and tooth decay, while consuming sorbitol or sucrose did not.[168]

In this intervention, patients were studied who had their normal saliva flow compromised because of radiation treatment for head and neck cancers. Individuals with no or little natural saliva are at greater risk of tooth decay. The results of this clinical trial clearly demonstrated that participants who had compromised salivary function and who ate natural honey had a significantly lower amount of Strep Mutans (a bacterium that causes tooth decay) than the control group.[169]

Of course, as with almost everything, there is good honey and bad honey. Processed or heated honey has lost most of its medicinal benefits. Honey that had anything added to it would not be my choice. The best honey to consume is locally raised, unfiltered, raw honey.

So, how much honey should you consume?

Many studies on humans suggest that the ideal amount of honey to consume per day for a 150-pound person is approximately 3-4 tablespoons.[170, 171] Some beneficial results have been recorded within an hour or two of ingestion.

Nuts and seeds

Nuts and seeds provide healthy fats and other nutrients, but they also contain anti-nutrients such as lectins and phytic acid. Many antinutrients may not be a problem; some are. (I discuss antinutrients in the next section, *U: UNDO the Damage*.)

Nuts and seeds have varying amounts of omega-6 to omega-3 ratios. A few nuts and seeds are OK, but eating them by the handful could be problematic. Be sure the nuts and seeds you consume are fresh because the polyunsaturated component in nuts and seeds can oxidize easily and become unhealthy.

Because of the antinutrients on the surface of most nuts and seeds, it is best to soak them six to twelve hours to remove these antinutrient molecules. Simply mix some sea salt in warm water and add the raw nuts and seeds to the water to soak. Then, strain and rinse them. You could eat them wet or allow them to dry for later use. A dehydrator is a perfect way to dry them. Or, you could place them on parchment paper on a cookie sheet in an oven at its lowest temperature until dried.

One of the healthiest nuts with a low level of polyunsaturated fat and high level of monounsaturated fat is the macadamia nut (fat content approximately 17% saturated fat, 81% monounsaturated fat, and 2% polyunsaturated fat with an omega-6 to omega-3 ratio of 6:1).

Following is a sampling of nuts and seeds and their fat breakdown[172]:

Nut	Sat. Fat	Mono. Fat	Poly. Fat	Omega-6: Omega-3
Almond	8%	66%	26%	28:1
Brazil	25%	41%	34%	1,142:1
Cashew	20%	60%	20%	48:1
Chia	11%	8%	81%	0.33:1
Flax Seed	9%	19%	72%	0.26:1
Hazelnut	7%	79%	14%	90:1
Macadamia	17%	81%	2%	6:1
Peanut (legume)	15%	52%	33%	5,162:1
Pecan	9%	59%	32%	21:1
Pine Nut	9%	32%	59%	300:1
Pistachio	13%	55%	32%	52:1
Pumpkin	20%	32%	48%	114:1
Sunflower	10%	40%	50%	312:1
Walnut	10%	14%	76%	4:1

Herbs and spices

Herbs and spices offer many nutrients even when used in small quantities. Not only do these make food tastier, they also are very healthy. Consider chili peppers, cocoa, sage, garlic, thyme, cinnamon, rosemary, turmeric, parsley, and oregano to name a few.[173]

Fermented foods

Our primal ancestors never knew about microbes. They occasionally ate foods that were rotting, but they were unaware of the bacterial process since microorganisms weren't discovered until the 17th century. The first recorded reference to fermented foods was about 8,000 years ago when grapes were fermented into wines in the Caucasus. Since then, societies learned that fermentation could allow foods to be preserved and eaten at a later date without rotting.

Fermented foods such as sauerkraut, kimchi, full-fat plain yogurt, full-fat plain kefir, other fermented vegetables, and kombucha (fermented tea) provide healthy bacteria that can support a healthy gut. Be sure these foods contain live cultures. If they have been pasteurized after the fermentation process, then the beneficial bacteria would have been destroyed. Include these healthy, live-culture, fermented choices with your meals as often as you can.

Homemade bone broth

Many chronic diseases appear to be rooted in an unbalanced mix of microorganisms in the digestive system because of a diet containing acellular carbohydrates, unhealthy fats, and other unhealthy elements. Various digestive problems have been helped with homemade bone broth[174].

The collagen found in bone broth helps to heal and seal the gut lining, and broth contains a variety of valuable nutrients in a form your body can easily absorb and use. They include but are not limited to:

- Calcium, phosphorus, and other minerals
- Silicon and other trace minerals
- Glucosamine and chondroitin sulfate
- Components of collagen and cartilage
- Components of bone and bone marrow
- Amino acids: proline, glycine, and glutamine

How to make the best broth

An efficient way to make homemade bone broth is to use a slow-cooker or crockpot. You can put a few basic ingredients into the pot, turn it on low heat, and in twenty-four to thirty-six hours it's done. You could make it faster in a pressure cooker. But, if you don't give the broth enough time, then you will not extract the nutrients that are so beneficial.

The more gelatinous the broth, the more nourishing it will tend to be. The collagen that leaches out of the bones when slow-cooked is one of the key ingredients that make broth so healing. You can make bone broth using whole organic chicken or just the feet, backs, or necks; whole fish or fish bones including the fish head, pork, or beef bones such as the marrowbones, oxtails, feet, or knuckles.

One of the most important aspects of the broth-making process is to use high-quality bones. Ideally, you'll want to use organically-raised animal bones--the younger the animal the better. An excellent animal bone choice would be veal bones, since they are very young when butchered. Use their femur and joint bones in a ratio of 1:1 for the best brew.

If you can't find a local source for organic bones, you could order them online. Otherwise, your best source might be from farmers at local farmers' markets. Many small farmers will raise their livestock according to organic principles even if their farm is not *USDA certified organic*, since certification is quite costly.

Another important part of the process I already mentioned is to cook the bones long enough to extract their nutrients. You could even reuse bones to make at least one more batch. Some people have suggested that you could reuse bones until they actually get soft. I personally am not sure how nutritionally beneficial the broth would be after the bones had been used for several brews.

The last important element that is necessary for success is to use *apple cider vinegar* or other type of vinegar in the broth ingredients to help chemically leach out the nutrients from the bones.

Use this broth for soups, stews, or drink it straight as any other cup of soup. If you are not going to use the broth in a few days, you should freeze it because of potential bacterial growth. I have included several recipes at the end of the book explaining not only how to make bone broth but also how to incorporate it into other recipes. (Bone Broth in Slow-Cooker, French Onion Oxtail Stew, Mushroom and Seaweed Soup, for instance.)

Clean water

Water is not nutrient-dense. However, water that is laden with unwanted chemicals could be bad. Our primal ancestors did not have filtered water, but their water did not have toxic substances as some of our drinking water has today. Therefore, filtered water will provide minimal toxic substances as well as necessary hydration. Recent evidence suggests that if you drink when you are thirsty, your body will have sufficient water intake. Usually 6-8 cups a day should be adequate. Adding a tablespoon or two of fresh lemon juice, lime juice, or apple cider vinegar to your water during the course of a day can help the acid quality in your stomach and detoxification. It also may prevent kidney stones and buildup of uric acid crystals.

Vitamin D

You've heard many times that exposure to the sun causes cancer. That's what everybody tells us. That may be true for repeated sunburn and overexposure. But, our bodies are designed to use the sun's UVB rays to make vitamin D in our skin through an efficient and natural way. We should not deny our bodies of what they require, but we need to be careful and not overdo it.

Vitamin D has been shown to be critical in many metabolic and physiologic processes. In the peer-reviewed literature, there have been several articles discussing Vitamin D and its relationship to gum disease.[175,176]

To become metabolically active, vitamin D that is produced on the skin from sun exposure is first converted in the liver to *calcidiol* [25(OH)D], which is clinically measured by the *25-Hydroxy Vitamin D* serum test. It is then further converted in the kidneys into the active form of vitamin D called *calcitriol* [1,25(OH)₂D].

Most people don't get enough vitamin D. It is estimated that 42% of the US population has a vitamin D deficiency with the highest rate seen in African Americans (82.1%), followed by Hispanics (69.2%).[177] Vitamin D deficiency is defined as a serum *25-Hydroxy Vitamin D* concentration of less than 20 ng/mL.

In a paper published in 2008, Bischoff-Ferrari suggested that an ideal serum level to help prevent cancer would be 36-48 ng/mL.[178] An extensive review of the literature published in 2015 by Robert Heaney, MD, suggested the ideal range for an individual would be 40-60 ng/mL.[179] The only way to know if you have a deficiency is to have a *25-Hydroxy Vitamin D* blood test done.

In 2013, Alshouibi et al showed that total daily vitamin D3 intake greater than 800 IU was associated with lower odds of severe periodontal disease relative to taking less than 400 IU/day. The authors reported that Vitamin D3 intake may protect against the progression of periodontal disease.[180]

In 2014, Martelli et al performed a literature search and determined that a decreased level of Vitamin D may increase the risk of developing periodontal disease by way of (1) an effect on bone mineral density or (2) other metabolic pathways such as those involved in immune response and chronic inflammation.[181]

Also in 2014, Andrukhov et al suggested that vitamin D might play an important role in the modulation of periodontal inflammation by way of the regulation of cytokine production by cells of the periodontal ligament.[182]

The amount of sun you need to stimulate Vitamin D production depends on the time of day, the season of the year, where you are in relation to the equator, the color of your skin, how old you are, and how much clothing you are wearing while in the sun. You also need to know how much Vitamin D is already in your body and how much you get from other sources such as foods or supplements.

The best way to manufacture vitamin D is to be in the sunshine. The next best way is to eat fatty fish such as wild caught salmon, pastured organ meats such as liver, and pastured egg yolks. The third way would be to take an appropriate dose of a vitamin D3 supplement.

It is important to note that vitamin D does not work by itself in the body. There is an important relationship between vitamin D and the bioavailability of various nutrients such as vitamins A and K₂, calcium, magnesium, zinc, boron, and others from the foods you consume in order for vitamin D to be effective.

To help determine how much sun you may require for your body, there is an app called DMinder[183] for smartphones and tablets that also helps track your exposure in the sun based on the variables I have described.

Bottom line: to assist in overall health and periodontal health, you might want to strive to maintain a serum level of approximately 50 ng/mL of *25-Hydroxy Vitamin D* obtained not only from the sun but also from a combination of nutrient-dense food choices and supplementation if necessary.

Supplements

In 2014, I wanted to learn how specific nutrient-dense foods might affect the progression of gum disease. I could not find any published research. So, I designed an in-office study of my own to find out. For the study, thirteen of my patients elected to take a blend of fermented cod liver oil with high vitamin butter, skate liver oil, and kelp powder (all in capsule form) for a period of thirty days. To be eligible for the study, all patients had to have bleeding gums and deep gum pockets. At the end of the study, there was a significant reduction both in bleeding gums and the depth of gum pockets.

I usually don't believe in supplements because our bodies were designed to be nourished from real foods found in nature rather than packaged substitutes. When you eat nutrient-dense foods, you'll rarely have a need for supplements.[184] However, the following supplements are unlike the packaged nutritional supplements with which you may be familiar.

Think of these as an extra-bump-up from the nutrient-dense foods I discussed above.

- Fermented cod-liver oil combined with high vitamin butter oil is anti-inflammatory and includes an abundance of naturally occurring fat-soluble vitamins A, D, E, and K among many other nutrients. Eating organ meats will give you what you need. However, if you need additional sources for these nutrients, you may want to look into products from Green Pasture.[185]

- Organic kelp powder and granules provide many trace minerals including iodine, which are synergistic with fat-soluble vitamins. If you include naturally occurring seaweeds (sea vegetables) in your diet, you'll be getting these important nutrients. However, if eating sea vegetables isn't part of your normal diet, these supplements could provide what you need in a natural composition. I use Maine Coast brand of organic kelp granules. It comes in a shaker-type container. If you want to take a capsule, I have used Oregon's Wild Harvest Organic Kelp Powder Caps with success.[186]

- Probiotics are healthy bacteria that help increase available bacteria in the gut. Good bacteria are easily consumed if you eat fermented foods as I described in the beginning of this chapter. If they are not available, then soil-based probiotics provide a variety of beneficial microorganisms that are difficult to get with a regular probiotic supplement. Usually, probiotics are not necessary to take over a long course of time. My favorite soil-based probiotic is Prescript-Assist®.[187]

- Prebiotics, which are soluble fibers, are important to feed your healthy gut microbiome. They are abundant in fruits and vegetables. An excellent additional source of a prebiotic is resistant starch. This is non-digestible by your gut but is food for healthy bacteria in your colon. It also is great to assist in intestinal motility for regular bowel movements. Start with only one teaspoon dissolved in water per day and gradually increase to as much as two to four tablespoons a day. If you take too much in the beginning, your body will overreact with gas, bloating, and diarrhea as the bad bacteria rebel, and you won't be saying good things about me if that happens! An excellent source is Bob's Red Mill Unmodified Potato Starch, which is readily available online or in most grocery stores.

Other supplements

I'd like to take a moment to discuss antioxidants because nearly everything you've heard about them may not be true!

Antioxidants are among the most popular *health-protecting supplements* sold worldwide without prescription. As a society, we think we need to purchase them in huge amounts in order to help rid our bodies of all those bad free radicals that are running around causing harm to our cells. But ongoing research[188] shows that "it ain't necessarily so."

Free radicals are molecules or atoms containing an unpaired electron. Unpaired electrons are hungry for another electron with which to pair up. Electrons want to exist in pairs. They are unstable until they get that additional electron from somewhere else so that they can be paired up again.

However, free radicals are naturally occurring byproducts of normal functions within the cells of our body. They are formed from the cell's use of oxygen to produce energy. In turn, these free radicals, in the form of *oxidative stress*, can signal the cell to create its own homemade antioxidants through the pathway of Nrf2[189]. Activation of Nrf2 can also be stimulated by various nutrients in foods, and this process is critical to our survival.

Antioxidants are molecules that are able to donate an electron to the free radical, thus stabilizing the free radical by giving it the extra electron to make a happy pair. If free radicals are unable to get their needed electrons from antioxidants, these radicals can cause damage to the body through *oxidative stress*, which is associated with ageing, heart failure, cancer, Alzheimer's, and many other health problems.

In the past, science has suggested that the more antioxidants we ingest, the less oxidative stress we have to endure. These antioxidants donate electrons to the free radicals and neutralize their potential damage. However, antioxidants themselves can become reactive (become a free radical themselves) after donating an electron to a free radical.

In the human body there are many varieties of antioxidants naturally present. As I mentioned, we produce them internally by stimulating the Nrf2 pathway. Also, our body can obtain antioxidants from nutrient-dense foods we ingest from a primal diet. The varieties of antioxidants in our system can buffer each other as they in turn give up electrons to newly formed free radical molecules.

As an example, one naturally occurring external source of antioxidants is chocolate. It contains more than 20 antioxidant flavonoids. Once you eat chocolate, its antioxidants have the ability to donate electrons to free radicals in the body. As one type of flavonoid gives up an electron to a free radical, this flavonoid is converted into a free radical itself and becomes reactive, but *less* so than the free radical to which it donated its electron. This reactive flavonoid then receives an electron from another type of flavonoid within the chocolate. This second flavonoid becomes reactive but, again, less so than the first flavonoid. This process continues with each successive flavonoid giving up an electron but becoming less reactive along the way. Eventually, the naturally occurring antioxidants in chocolate (in this example) decrease the damage of free radicals in our body.

A problem occurs when we take a high-dose antioxidant supplement. For example, taking a high-dose vitamin C supplement provides only one form of antioxidant. There are no other antioxidants in this supplement to offer the protective *give and take* by providing extra electrons. The end result could be an abundance of antioxidant molecules of vitamin C that are now free radicals themselves. They have become highly reactive with no means of neutralizing themselves. This creates more *oxidative stress*.

The bottom line is to help your body produce its own antioxidants as necessary and to utilize the antioxidants supplied in nutrient-dense foods. Taking doses of antioxidant supplements could prove unhealthy, resulting in more oxidative stress than you had before! Eating a nutrient-dense diet such as the primal diet not only could promote activation of the Nrf2 pathway but also could provide numerous varieties of beneficial antioxidants for your cells.

U - UNDO the damage

Our body is amazingly resilient. It can cope with a great deal of insult. However, insults build over time, and the cumulative effects can become hazardous to your health. These insults might originate:

- With foods that have not been digested properly and seeped into our bloodstream.
- As a result of environmental toxic substances that accumulated in our tissues.
- From psychological stress or other physical and chemical stresses.
- As some invading foreign body, such as a splinter or an improperly fitting dental filling leaking mercury into the system.

This is important, and you must understand it thoroughly: Problems do not become serious overnight. They creep up slowly without warning. It might take decades for individual cellular dysfunction to manifest itself into clinical and obvious symptoms. When dysfunction does manifest itself, the problem may seem to have happened suddenly. *But it just ain't so!*

Here is a typical scenario:

You've been eating a Standard American Diet (SAD) consisting of unhealthy fats, acellular carbs, minimal vegetables, and processed foods for years without any obvious problems. In your teens and then in your twenties, nothing seemed to be wrong with your weight or your health except a little gum bleeding. Then "all of a sudden" in your thirties you developed a little "belly" and maybe a slightly higher blood pressure. You also noticed your blood sugar was a little higher than it used to be, and maybe there was still occasional gum bleeding. In your forties you developed other signs and symptoms of chronic disease such as joint problems, maybe stomach distress, maybe skin issues, possibly a little brain fog. Perhaps the gum bleeding was not so much of a problem, but some of your teeth were starting to get sensitive and loose. The subtle but obvious symptoms you began to notice in your forties all started with the cellular damage that began decades before. Chronic disease doesn't happen overnight. Decades might have passed before these outward manifestations became obvious.

Undoing the damage requires each of us to remove as many of the stresses on our body as possible. We live in a world that will not allow us to eliminate all the potential external and internal insults we face each day. Nor can we completely remove all the insults we have already sustained. But, we should strive to do our best.

A good part of the damage to our body comes from eating the wrong things (and, conversely, not eating the right things). Later in this chapter I will discuss other insults that affect our lives.

Eating the wrong things
The eating style and physical lifestyle I recommend are based on human evolution--sometimes known as the Paleo Lifestyle, Ancestral Lifestyle, or Primal Lifestyle. They basically are all the same.

Below are some of the foods that our ancestors never ate because most of these didn't exist over the 2.5 million years of human evolution. Our bodies were never designed to ingest and digest these foods. In some way or another, they disrupt the normal digestion and absorption processes. Some of these foods our bodies may tolerate. However, our bodies absolutely *require* none of them; all the nutrients our bodies need are more easily obtained from the nutrient-dense foods discussed in the previous chapter. The three categories of foods that are most damaging to overall health are dense acellular carbohydrates, unhealthy fats, and antinutrients.

- *Dense acellular carbs* must be eliminated, not merely reduced! Even small amounts have been shown to cause damage within our cells. Dense acellular carbohydrates rarely exist in nature, the vast majority being manmade. Processed grain and refined sugar products are examples of acellular carbohydrates. Their carbohydrate density is also counterproductive to weight maintenance.

- *Unhealthy fats and oils* are those in the polyunsaturated fat category that are chemically and biologically damaging to our cells. These oils are easily oxidized and can confuse and poison our normal metabolism. They create problems that may compound and become evident many years later. The problems include damaged cell membranes, damaged DNA/RNA strands, and damaged blood vessels. Also, saturated fats from animals that have been fed grains or unnatural food products and have been given chemicals and hormones will have unhealthy elements in their fat that should be avoided. All manmade trans fats are highly toxic to our body.

- *Antinutrients*[190] are compounds that have the potential to interfere with the absorption of necessary nutrients by our body. They actually are important defense mechanisms for plants that help protect plants from predators. There are many types of antinutrients, but the major categories I will discuss are lectins, phytic acids, and oxalates. Some of them are easy to remove; some of them are impossible to remove; some of them may be beneficial for us. Many foods contain these compounds, but the foods that have the highest concentration of antinutrients are grains, legumes, nuts, and seeds.

  o Lectins are proteins that can attach to the sugars in cell membranes. In the intestine, they cause damage to the gut lining, improper absorption of nutrients, and tears in the intestinal wall causing leakage into the bloodstream. Once in the bloodstream, they create inflammation that can affect the entire body. These can be the most dangerous of the antinutrients because some of them are difficult or impossible to eliminate through soaking and cooking. Gluten is the best-known lectin, but non-gluten grains contain other lectins that also may be problematic.

o   Phytic acids appear in many foods. Nuts, seeds, beans/legumes, and grains store phosphorus as phytic acid. When phytic acid is bound to a mineral in the seed, it's known as phytate. Phytic acids bind to minerals (especially zinc, iron, magnesium, copper, and calcium) in the foods that we are eating and prevent them from being absorbed through the small intestine. Phytic acid can also interfere with digestive enzymes and can irritate the gut. Generally, damaging phytic acid can be eliminated from nuts and seeds by simply soaking them properly. The major problem for our bodies is the quantity of phytic acid consumed and not merely the consumption, itself. Here, moderation is key.

o   Oxalates appear in raw vegetables such as kale, chard, and spinach and can bind to calcium. Oxalates in large quantities on a daily basis can be damaging to our bodies. In moderation they do not seem to be a general problem. Most can be reduced significantly through cooking.

Let's talk

Many experts suggest that some of the foods I list below can be prepared in various ways to make them less harmful. That is definitely true. If you were set on eating specific foods that would be harmful if not prepared expertly, you could make the effort to prepare those foods the proper way. But, my question to you is, *Why?* Why go to the trouble of attempting to remove bad compounds from specific foods when all the nutrition you need to survive and thrive is found in the foods I described in the last chapter?

With that said, here are the foods that I believe you should avoid for all the right reasons:

Modern grains and grain products, also known as cereal grains, can create inflammation and a leaky gut, through which undigested foods and bad bacteria can leak into the bloodstream. Not good! This creates a cascade of events that can cause various chronic diseases and obesity. Grains also encourage the overgrowth of unhealthy bacteria in the gut, which never evolved to digest grains completely. An abundance of unhealthy bacteria in the gut means unhealthy bacteria in the mouth. Grains need to be eliminated from our diets.

Pseudograins are foods that resemble cereal grains. Cereal grains are the seeds of grasses. In contrast, pseudograins are the seeds of broadleaf plants. The three major pseudograins are amaranth, buckwheat, and quinoa. These pseudograins generally are less troublesome than cereal grains, but they still contain lectins, phytates, and other antinutrients that may be bothersome for some people. Pseudograins, just the same as cereal grains, also contain an abundance of carbohydrates that can interfere with maintenance of healthy body weight. Pseudograins are not essential for health.

Unnatural sugars contribute to unhealthy bacteria and chronic diseases just the way grains do. From a dental standpoint, sugars are fermentable carbohydrates that feed unhealthy oral bacteria, which cause dental decay and gum disease. All added sugars such as fructose, agave, and high fructose corn syrup, should be avoided. Also, limit the amount of fruits you eat because of the high fructose content. As I described in the section "G: Give yourself nutrient-dense nourishment," raw honey has a unique place in the health of our bodies.

Artificial sweeteners also fall into this category of foods to avoid. When you eat something sweet, your brain releases dopamine, which activates your brain's reward center. The appetite-regulating hormone leptin is also released, which eventually informs your brain that you are "full" once a certain amount of nutrients have been ingested. However, when you consume something that tastes sweet but *doesn't* contain any nutrients, your brain's pleasure pathway still gets activated by the sweet taste, but there's nothing to deactivate it, since the nutrients never arrive. Artificial sweeteners are notorious for tricking your body into thinking it's going to receive sugar (a carbohydrate nutrient), but when the sugar doesn't come, your body continues to signal that it needs more, which results in carb cravings. Besides worsening insulin sensitivity, damaging the gut microbiome, and promoting weight gain[191], artificial sweeteners also promote other health problems such as cardiovascular disease and stroke.[192]

Unhealthy fats and oils (such as canola oil, sunflower oil, soybean oil, corn oil, and safflower oil) are unstable and break down easily as a result of commercial processing and normal cooking. These are polyunsaturated oils that are easily reactive with oxygen, which causes oxidation making these fats inflammatory and unstable. Oxidation is analogous to the chemical reaction between oxygen and iron in the presence of moisture to form rust. Ingestion of these oils damages metabolic processes causing harm to individual cells. These oils also can become incorporated into the cells' membranes further compromising the health and function of cells.

Another unhealthy fat group is chemically altered trans fats and partially hydrogenated fats. These are man-made to attempt to make fats more shelf-stable and solid, but these fats are toxic to the body.

Also to be avoided are the saturated fats from animals that have been fed grains or unnatural feed products, or have been injected with hormones, antibiotics, or other chemical substances.

All unhealthy fats and oils need to be avoided.

Processed foods contain too many acellular carbohydrates, unhealthy fats, and an excess of unhealthy salt. They also contain various chemicals, which attempt to add back nutrients and to help food maintain a longer shelf life. Many of these additives are toxic. Basically, processed foods are foods that have been commercially prepared, packaged with various labels, and line the shelves of grocery store aisles. Usually, unprocessed foods line the periphery of the grocery stores where you might find fresh animal products, fruits, and vegetables. A general rule of thumb (but not etched in stone) would be to shop the periphery of the grocery store and not the aisles of the grocery store, where the packaged processed foods reside. Processed foods should be avoided.

Legumes have antinutrients such as lectins and phytic acid that potentially irritate the intestinal lining and prevent proper absorption of many minerals. Legumes are not essential for health, and their nutrients can be obtained from more healthy selections discussed in the previous chapter. Legumes include most beans, peas, lentils, soy, and peanuts.

Commercially available soy and peanuts should always be avoided because cooking cannot destroy peanuts' antinutrients, and soy contains phytoestrogens and trypsin inhibitors. The phytoestrogens may confuse the body into thinking it is real estrogen, and the trypsin inhibitors can interfere with normal protein digestion.

However, soaking other beans, peas, and lentils for 8-12 hours and cooking them long enough to reduce the harmful level of antinutrients are methods that *may* make these legumes less harmful.

Milk products from commercially raised cattle are generally unhealthy. Grain-fed cows' milk that is pasteurized and homogenized is considered "dead." The processes of pasteurization and homogenization destroy beneficial fats, bacteria, enzymes, and proteins in the milk. In addition, the lectins from grain feed that are ingested by cattle get into their milk and then into our cells. Also, the antibiotics and hormones administered to these cattle to "keep them healthy" are transferred by way of their milk into us. The only milk products I recommend are non-homogenized, raw milk and its products sourced from grass-fed/grass-finished pastured cows or goats that have never been exposed to any antibiotics, hormones, or other chemicals. You can find sources of raw milk products located in your zip code area at www.realmilk.com.

Other insults to our bodies

Bad foods are a problem that can be avoided. You simply need to make the choice to eliminate them. Other insults to our body also should be eliminated or reduced to improve the health of our cells. Everything boils down to the health of each cell. We need to do whatever it takes to make our cells function as they were intended.

After all, you take your car to be serviced regularly so that the engine purrs like a kitten, it's safe to drive, and it reliably transports you from place to place. Why not treat your body with the same respect and responsibility? That means giving your cells what they need and removing what they don't.

Stress!

And let's not forget about stress. It can kill you. Or it can be life-saving. It runs the gamut.

Stress takes many forms. It can take the form of chemical insults (such as insecticides or heavy metals) or physical trauma (such as excessive exercise or an accident). It can be biological in origin (such as oxidative stress) or psychological (such as emotional or mental strain).

The bodily damage from stress is not necessarily obvious at first. Stress builds up over time until the proverbial *straw that breaks the camel's back*.

As various stressors affect the body, healthy immune and detoxification systems deal with them. But, as event after event occurs, stress can create a greater and greater load. At some point in time, the total stress load could overpower the natural systems that were designed to deal with it. Then clinical manifestations might raise their ugly heads to become problems.

Psychological stress is a state of mental or emotional strain or tension resulting from adverse or very demanding circumstances. It can be acute and short lived or chronic and reoccurring.

A recent paper written by Barry Oken, et al, was published in April 2015, titled, *A Systems Approach to Stress, Stressors and Resilience in Humans*.[193] In the *Introduction* section of the paper, the authors discussed several telling factors: A recent survey indicated that 25% of Americans reported high stress and 50% identified a major stressful event during the previous year. Chronic psychological stress might increase the risk of health problems and could contribute to cardiovascular problems as well as neurologic and psychiatric diseases such as epilepsy, Parkinson's disease, multiple sclerosis, eating disorders, addictions, post-traumatic stress disorder (PTSD), and sleep difficulties.

In addition stress affects the gut microbiome, the immune system, and even the mouth[194]. When stress occurs, the human body reacts. Nerves and organs release chemicals and hormones during stressful times, and these biological substances prepare the body either to face the actual or perceived threat or to flee for safety (the "fight or flight" syndrome).

Observe yourself. When you face a dangerous situation, your pulse quickens; you breathe faster; and your muscles tense. Your brain begins to use more oxygen and to increase activity--all these functions are aimed at survival. In the short term, stress can *boost* the immune system.

However, with chronic stress that occurs repeatedly, these same chemicals and hormones that are life-saving in short bursts can suppress functions that aren't needed for immediate survival. Your immune system goes into a slowdown mode. Your digestive and excretory systems slow down, and your reproductive systems may actually shut down totally. Once the threat has passed, other body systems act to restore normal functioning. Clinical problems occur if the stress remains constant or if the stress response continues even after the danger has passed.

Everybody has stress in his or her life. Stress is normal. As a matter of fact, stress has many positive effects. In its acute state, stress is necessary for individuals to cope with the challenges of everyday life. As I suggested, if an event occurred that threatened your life, your immediate reaction to this stressor would activate your body's defense mechanisms to either fight off the threat or run away from it. This stress response could be life-saving. In primal days, when a ferocious animal was a threat, the stress response would have caused an individual to fight the animal or flee from the danger.

However, when stress begins to become chronic, lasting for long periods of time or being repeated often, it becomes biologically destructive. Stress can consume one's life and change it from exciting and hopeful to uninteresting and foreboding. All parts of the body can be victimized by chronic stress. Modern day stresses such as financial concerns, fear of failure, and abusive relationships may become chronic. Since our bodies deal with stress as *life-or-death* situations, when stress happens continuously, our bodies break down.

Biologically, stress may affect the mouth by constricting blood vessels; exaggerating the reaction of the immune system; disrupting the healthy equilibrium of the gut and mouth bacteria; decreasing saliva flow, and suppressing appetite.

As stress affects the immune system, areas of the mouth that may be susceptible could break down. Various biological chemicals in the mucosal tissues of the mouth may become affected, which can result in lesions and eruptions of these tissues. In the end, the result of psychological stress could create damage in the mouth. [195,196,197,198,199]

Some of the manifestations of stress occur in the soft tissues of the mouth, and examples might be *aphthous ulcers* and periodontal disease.

Total stress load

Total stress load is demanding on a cellular level and must be reduced. Stress can build internally from *emotional stresses*, but they can also stem from *physical* and *chemical stresses*. *Dental problems* can also cause the body stress. All these can accumulate over time and become detrimental to overall health. What you can avoid completely, you should avoid. What you can reduce, you should reduce. Let's take a closer look at the three major types of stress.

Emotional stresses can come about as a result of how you deal with life itself, how you perceive yourself in society, or how you react mentally to potentially harmful situations.

Physical stresses can result from over-exercising. [200] Over-exercising increases the production of free radicals, which are produced as oxygen is used for energy production in muscle contractions. This enhanced free radical generation causes oxidative damage to muscles and other tissues and causes damage to cellular membranes leading to chronic, systemic inflammation. Chronic inflammation is implicated in diseases such as cancer, heart disease, strokes, MS, Alzheimer's, Parkinson's, premature aging, and almost any other debilitating, degenerative condition you can name. In the next chapter, I'll describe some healthy exercise routines that don't take much time, provide significant benefits, and reduce excess and chronic physical stress.

Chemical stresses could be the result of toxic elements in foods, bacterial infections, environmental toxic substances, and toxic products placed in your mouth by your dentist.

- Toxic elements in food take the form of food coloring, preservatives, synthetic ingredients, unnatural fats and oils, and other chemical additives. Read the ingredient label on the food package! If the words are more than two syllables long or too scientific, those ingredients are probably unhealthy for you.
- Bacterial infections produce various byproducts from the bacteria as well as from the body's defense mechanisms that could be toxic to your cells. Gum infections fit this category. If an infection exists, it needs to be identified and treated by an appropriate healthcare professional.
- Environmental toxic substances are abundant and include aluminum in antiperspirants, heavy metals in water and other foods, and insecticides and cleaning chemicals inside and outside your home. A solution is to use deodorants that don't have aluminum as an ingredient; to use filtered water for drinking and cooking; and investigate non-chemical methods to use around your home.
- Some materials that are used in dentistry also could be toxic to your body. Examples would be mercury in "silver fillings"; some metals or plastics incorporated into tooth replacements such as crowns, bridges, implants, and partials; some materials used in plastic appliances placed in the mouth; some composite resins used to restore decaying teeth; and some sealants that are placed on a tooth's chewing surface to seal off small grooves in those surfaces where bacteria could lodge.

Your body is designed to remove most toxic substances with which you come in contact--especially if they are intermittent. Detoxification is mainly performed by your liver. Therefore, it is critical to provide the nutrients necessary to maintain a healthy functioning liver. The healthy food choices in the previous chapter give your body the nutrients to successfully manage most toxic loads. Healthier lifestyle choices can avoid and eliminate most other stressors. But, if you are bombarded with toxic substances on a regular basis and your body gets backlogged in the detoxification process, you may need more help in ridding these from your tissues. A Functional Medicine Practitioner treating these issues could be the person to see in order to delve deeper into the cellular problems and their resolutions.

Toxic materials placed in your mouth by a dentist are a different matter because they are not intermittent. They stay in the materials that stay in your mouth. Some toxic elements may stay in the material itself and not leach out to harm you. Some materials may be harmful to some people who are sensitive to them while other people will not have a reaction. Other materials are harmful only when they reach a certain concentration or begin to accumulate in your body because of continuous exposure.

There are steps you can take to avoid or limit these exposures to dental toxic material. You need to be proactive when seeing your dentist. Fluoride, mercury, bisphenol-A (BPA), methyl methacrylate, and some other substances may be toxic elements to your body. You should question your dentist about any material he or she plans to put into your mouth. There are blood tests evaluated by various labs to see if you are potentially sensitive to certain materials used in dental materials. Your dentist could have you go to a facility to have blood drawn, which would then be submitted to specific labs to determine if you might be sensitive to particular materials to be used in your mouth.

Two such laboratories that provide these tests are Clifford Consulting Laboratory[201] and Biocomp Laboratories.[202]

Another test that is unique is the Melisa test[203], which shows sensitivity to titanium. However, you need to be aware that these tests may not always be conclusive. They may show false negatives (which means the test says you are not sensitive but you actually are) or false positives (which means that the test says you are sensitive but you actually *aren't*).

A dental problem can be similar to a splinter in your finger that never gets removed. The longer it stays in place, the more damage it can do to the surrounding tissues. All of the following problems may not cause any discomfort initially. But, these problems could cause swelling, spread of infection, and pain if not treated appropriately. They may cause difficulty in chewing your food. Remember, the natural process of digestion begins in the mouth. If food cannot be broken down properly in the mouth, part of the digestion process could be compromised.

- *Broken or Infected Teeth*: These allow bacteria to seep into microscopic crevices and break down the tooth surfaces as well as infect the gum and bone tissues. Deeper infection could cause the nerve of the tooth to die, creating an abscess.

- *Poor Dentistry*: Sometimes a filling or crown is not made to fit ideally in the mouth. A poorly designed filling or crown could cause bite problems damaging the actual tooth itself, the bone around the tooth root, or the jaw joint and the muscles of the jaw.

- *Broken Fillings*: These could cause the same effects as a broken or infected tooth.

- *Splinters Under Gum*: Generally these are calcified remnants of bacteria attached to the roots of teeth much the same way barnacles would attach to the bottom of a boat that sits in the water. They are called calculus or tartar. These are irritants to the surrounding gum and bone and can encourage further progression of an infection until they are removed.

- *Infections Inside Tooth (necrotic teeth)*: The nerve that lives inside the canal of a tooth root is positioned like the carbon in the center of a pencil. If this dies or becomes infected, its infection would push out of the tooth at the base of the root (like the pencil point at the writing tip of a pencil). The infection could then spread into the surrounding bone causing pain and swelling and actually spreading to other parts of the body.

- *Hopelessly Compromised Teeth*: If a tooth becomes damaged in such a way that it can't be repaired, it should be removed or further infection or damage could occur.
- *Forces Creating Unhealthy Pressures on Teeth*: If one tooth hits another tooth for whatever reason and in such a way as to wiggle that other tooth, then the heavy pressure or forces would need to be smoothed down to eliminate rocking of the tooth. Otherwise, the constant unnatural pressures could crack the tooth or damage the surrounding bone or the jaw muscles.
- *Improper Alignment of Teeth:* Poor alignment of teeth can be corrected by an orthodontist (a dental specialist that helps to move teeth using bands and wires or other appliances to get a healthier biting relationship). This could help prevent future chewing or jaw problems.
- *Other Infections or Damage to Gum, Teeth, Bone, Jaw Joint, or Muscles of Mastication*: A thorough examination by a well-trained dental practitioner should uncover other potential insults that may be occurring in your mouth causing unforeseen problems. A thorough evaluation will take more than a ten-minute exam. For my patients, I spend an hour doing a thorough mouth examination.

M - MASTER methods of maintenance

Each cell in your body is critical. The previous chapters should have encouraged you to make the necessary changes in your eating lifestyle to accomplish this.

To me, the perfect life would be full of the things that I wanted to do and that made me happy. Whatever difficult situations came my way, and there inevitably would be some that were extremely challenging, I would want to be able to deal with them and move on. I would want to spend quality time with those I love and cherish. I would want to be able to physically and mentally move into my senior years, aging graciously without chronic degenerative diseases that could decrease the quality of my life for decades. And then, as everyone would eventually experience at some endpoint, I would die.

The quality of my life means more to me than the quantity of my years.

So, here are some of the methods I have researched to assist in maintaining the highest quality of life for me. These may work for you. I am not one for going crazy implementing weird science and spending an enormous sum of money to purchase the next unique gizmo to make something more perfect. I want *simple*. I want to do things for myself and to myself that don't require a high cost or unreasonable time. I also want to make what I am doing easily repeatable over time. I believe that mastering these methods will go a long way to reach my goal of health. Let's start with the mouth and end with the total body.

Maintain a healthy mouth

Over the years, how many ways have you been told how to clean your mouth? For me, different dentists showed me different things when I was a kid; then different dental instructors told me different things while I was in dental school; and now, the marketing media all around us are screaming conflicting ways to make our mouths healthy. How do you sift through all of this stuff? Here is what should be appropriate for almost everyone.

- Coconut oil is anti-bacterial, anti-viral, and anti-fungal due mostly to its lauric acid content. It is solid at room temperature but liquid above 75°F. Interestingly, it can be used as a very effective mouth rinse (called "coconut oil pulling"), but you should use it only occasionally. Antimicrobial mouthwashes used regularly could damage healthy bacteria throughout your mouth that could cause unhealthy problems. To use it, place a teaspoon of coconut oil in your mouth; it will liquefy quickly. Swish for a few minutes and then spit it out into a napkin and not into the sink, where it could clog the pipes. Then, rinse with water. The science suggests that rinsing with coconut oil may be as effective as using chlorhexidine [204], a prescription mouthwash used to kill harmful bacteria. Just make sure you don't use the coconut oil on a regular basis because it may kill off the beneficial bacteria in your mouth.

- Two electric toothbrushes that I like are the Sonicare® rechargeable toothbrushes [205] and the OralB® Electric toothbrushes[206]. Electric brushes are so much more efficient than a regular manual toothbrush. I only like the ones that sit in a cradle and plug into the electric outlet. The replaceable battery types don't provide adequate torque for the bristles to function effectively in my opinion. To brush your teeth and gums with an electric toothbrush, dip the bristles of the brush first into coconut oil and then into baking soda. (In my bathroom, I have a small jar of coconut oil and a small jar of baking soda.) Place the brush into the space between the teeth and gum on the cheek side and then the tongue side of the teeth. Don't turn the brush "on" until the bristles are positioned at the gum line. Once the brush is turned "on," keep your lips closed as much as possible. You will still drool, so bend over your sink bowl. The idea is to let the soft bristles wiggle and clean into the gum space between the gum and the tooth just as you might visualize how you would clean the angle where the wall meets the floor with a scrub brush. Ideally, brush first thing in the morning and last thing before bed.

- To clean between the teeth, dental floss works well. In addition, you can clean between the teeth with a tiny-bristle brush that cleans the "in between" tooth surfaces like a bottlebrush cleans the inside of a bottle. Two popular types by the same company are the Soft-Picks® and the Proxabrush® [207]. Ideally, when you clean with the electric toothbrush, you also should clean between the teeth.

- Have professional cleanings with a hygienist on a regular basis based on your individual needs and not upon an arbitrary frequency.

- Brush your tongue.[208] An effective way is to use a teaspoon. This process will remove the odor-forming bacteria and some of the food remnants that play havoc with bad breath. Place the inverted teaspoon as far back as is comfortable on the upper side of your tongue. Then, gently glide the teaspoon forward, removing the bacterial film and microscopic food particles. Repeat this two to three times, and then wash off the teaspoon. Perform this tongue-cleaning method in the morning and then in the evening before bed.

Maintain a physically active body

Let's change gears and talk about the rest of the body.

Approximately 80% of your body's composition is based on the foods you consume. I already have suggested the foods that should be included, the ones that should be eliminated, and some possible supplements that have merit. Here is the rest of the story. And more...

Sun Exposure is necessary for your body to produce Vitamin D on your skin. As I discussed earlier, the proper exposure will not produce sunburn. The time in the sun is based on the time of day, the season of the year, where you are in relation to the equator, the color of your skin, how old you are, how much clothing you are wearing while in the sun, and how much Vitamin D you get from other sources such as foods or supplements.

I personally use DMinder[209], the app I suggested earlier, for my iPhone. I input my age, the last lab result of my *25-Hydroxy D* blood test, the nutrient-dense foods I eat that provide vitamin D, and how much clothing I wear. I take a picture of my face so that the app knows my skin tone. The app uses its built-in GPS to determine my location and the angle of the sun. It will use all this information to tell me how long I need to stay in the sun at that moment to reach my goal for vitamin D.

Caveat! Before engaging in any exercise routine, make sure you are physically capable of doing these exercises. You may need to consult your physician before you attempt the exercises I describe below.

Aerobic Exercise for about 2 hours a week helps burn fat and stabilize hormones. Exercise also has been shown to increase the growth of new brain cells in rats that have been given LPS, which normally would inhibit brain cell growth.[210]

Aerobic exercises should be performed at 55% to 75% of your estimated maximum heart rate, which is determined by this formula: 208 minus (your age x 0.7). As an example, if you were 50 years old, then your maximum heart rate would be 208 minus 35, or 173. Your aerobic routine should be performed between a heart rate of 95 (i.e. 55% of 173) beats per minute and 130 (i.e. 75% of 173) beats per minute. If you go below 95, there will be minimal exercise benefit; if you go above 130, the exercise becomes anaerobic, not what you want to do for an aerobic workout. Adequate rest between exercises is critical for healthy results. There are various wristbands or chest bands that will monitor your heart rate. It would not be practical to take your heart rate manually while exercising.

An exercise that I love is to ride my Trikke®[211] outdoors. For me, it's great exercise and great fun. I ride my Trikke® on the weekend first thing in the morning for about forty minutes unless the weather dictates otherwise.

Brief and intense strength training builds muscle strength and improves hormone efficiency that allows your body to function optimally and increase metabolism. Science has shown that doing four simple movements taking as little as ten to twenty minutes twice a week can get your body in shape. These movements are pull-ups, pushups, squats, and planks.

I do these four movements in the privacy and comfort of my home once or twice a week. I purchased a pull-up bar online and attached it to the doorframe of my bedroom. Here is an online source that reviews various pull up bars.[212] The squats, pushups, and planks require no equipment, only motivation. There are great videos demonstrating these movements on YouTube by Mark Sisson. The series is worth viewing: pull-ups[213], pushups[214], squats[215], and plank[216].

High intensity interval training is the ultimate beneficial exercise for your heart, your muscles, your hormones, and your weight. You could perform this once a week for ten to twenty minutes in total. You would start with a warm up of one to two minutes. Each cycle might consist of (1) seven to thirty seconds of all-out-to-exhaustion pedaling on a recumbent bike or sprinting outside, and (2) rest for about ninety seconds to regain your normal breath. This cycle should be repeated for two to eight times. Then, finish with a one- to two-minute cool down.

I use a Nordic Track Classic Pro Skier®[217], a cross-country ski machine that is set up in my spare bedroom. Usually I use it once a week for four to six cycles depending how I feel that day. I warm up by skiing at a slow pace for two minutes. Then, I "ski" at the fastest speed I can muster for twenty-five seconds, and then rest for ninety seconds. That completes one cycle, which I will repeat until done.

Non-exercise movement is just walking or moving about. Your goal should be to take approximately 10,000 steps a day. A pedometer is best to register these steps. Today, pedometers can be carried in your pocket, worn around your waist or wrist, or even worn around your neck. Here is an online review of various pedometers.[218] On average, walking about one mile is equivalent to 2,000 steps.

At first, I used a simple pedometer to determine how many steps I was getting into my day. You may be surprised (as I was) as to how few you are walking. Now I know how much I need to move to get my 10,000 or so steps into my daily routine. I am not always successful with my goal of 10,000 steps per day, but I do my best to be on target. Three mornings a week I am able to start my day by walking three miles in my neighborhood. This walk jump-starts my day with about 6,000 steps.

Standing rather than sitting has recently been shown to be important for overall health and for the health of your joints and stabilizing muscles. It has been postulated that sitting most of the day may be as unhealthy as smoking[219].

This has been difficult for me since treating patients in a dental office requires quite a bit of sitting. I try to stand as much as possible, and I use a standup desk while at home on my computer or while doing most anything I once did at my sitting desk.

Restorative sleep is not actually physical activity but rather physical inactivity. Sleep is critical to maintain normal hormonal repair in your body. But restorative sleep is not haphazard; it should be based on the natural circadian rhythm that is a result of the sun rising and setting at different times in the year. On average, it is best to get at least seven to eight hours of sleep each night, starting from the hours of 9-11 p.m. in a dark, cool setting.

I've done some research and experimented with my own sleep habits. Here are my thoughts on how to get to sleep, how to stay asleep, and how to wake up naturally:

- When the sun rises, it stimulates biochemicals in your body to get you up in the morning. When the sun sets, the lack of light stimulates biochemicals to make you sleepy. Therefore, it is important to have no light in your bedroom when you are ready for sleep. For a good night's sleep, make your bedroom dark, quiet, and temperature cool.
- Coffee and caffeine containing foods work on your central nervous system and prevent your brain from slowing down. Caffeine will keep you awake. Consequently, you don't want to drink coffee or eat foods containing caffeine shortly before bedtime. Here is an interesting video on YouTube® that explains how caffeine affects your body[220].
- Healthy root carbs can increase the production of melatonin, which is a hormone that is important to make you sleepy, while not creating a spike in blood sugar. An example of a healthy carb that can help you fall asleep is a

sweet potato. You could eat it with your dinner or as a snack before bedtime.

- If your last meal of the day is more than 3 hours before bedtime, you could have a blood sugar imbalance while asleep that could wake you up in the middle of the night. To stay asleep, try to eat your dinner no more than 3 hours before bedtime. It should consist of a balance of foods including protein, healthy carbohydrates, and healthy fats. This should help maintain proper blood sugar balance during your sleep cycle.

- Light will stimulate you to wake up. Natural sunlight coming into your bedroom will help you wake up naturally. Alternatively, an alarm clock using light to slowly illuminate the room, rather than using loud alarming sounds, can help you wake naturally. You could find many models online by Googling "sunrise alarm clocks."

There they are--five natural ways to get a good night's sleep that can be restorative for your whole body. Try my ideas, and get the sleep you need--naturally.

I personally get up early to start my day, so my bedtime usually is around 9 p.m. The lights are out, the room is cool, and it's quiet. I will wake about 4:30 a.m. to start my day on weekdays, and I am usually up by 6:00 a.m. on weekends.

Intermittent fasting improves overall physical health. [221] It improves insulin sensitivity, reduces oxidative stress, and increases your capacity to resist stress, disease, and aging. It is one of the most powerful means to shed excess weight and reduce your risk of chronic diseases once you have been successful at removing the bad foods and replacing them with nutrient-dense choices.

Intermittent fasting is *scheduled eating*. The best method I have found is to fast most days by restricting my eating from 11 a.m. to

7 p.m. I skip breakfast and make lunch my first meal of the day. This equals a fast of sixteen hours.

Stress-reducing techniques

Easier said than done! I've been there; I know. Psychological stresses affect your adrenal glands, thyroid gland, immune system, gut issues, and a host of other biological systems.

What really works for psychological stress? What has been proven to de-stress your stress without drugging you up? Here are 11 proven ideas, which are great starting points:

1. **Be present.** It boils down to one-on-one. Focus on the moment--not on the past or on the future--just on the moment. For example, if you have an important task you need to accomplish, you can stress out because you think there are a million other things waiting to be done. Or you can be present and focus completely on that task. Be present one-on-one--you and that one task. When you're done, you can move on to the next task. Then practice, practice, practice until "being present" becomes a habit.

2. **Just say, "NO!"** If you are stressed because you feel forced to do more than you physically and emotionally want to handle, then don't. Just say, "No!" Limit and prioritize your time to do those things you want and need to do.

3. **Avoid those people who stress you out.** There may be some people that put pressures on you, and these people may not be important in your life. If this is the case, then avoid them.

4. **Reduce your dependence on the news.** Constant news on TV and other media can be upsetting and depressing. If these sources create undue stress, then stop watching or listening to them. Get the news you need, but don't inundate yourself with it.

5. **Give up on pointless arguments.** You don't have to win every battle. You don't have to compromise your morals or ethics either, but you could assume *enough is enough* and just move on.

6. **Reframe situations that stress you.** Try to place situations in a different context. For example, if you're stuck in traffic, you might be able to listen to a podcast that you were planning to do later on, or you could just use this precious time to decompress or think through some of the priorities you have scheduled for the rest of your day.

7. **Lower your expectations and standards where possible.** You don't have to be 100% successful with every task. Sometimes 80% is good enough. When it is not, then strive for the remaining 20%.

8. **Realize things are what they are.** There are things you can't change. However, you don't have to compromise with those things you can and want to change.

9. **Discover gratitude.** Be thankful for the loved ones in your life and for those positive things you have accomplished in your life. You may want to keep a journal each day where you list two or three things you did that day that you're grateful for and how your actions may have contributed to those.

10. **Experience empathy for yourself and for others.** You will learn compassion for yourself, and you will better understand what affects others.

11. Explore and practice specific stress management practices. Here are a few:

    a. **Meditation:** It is not as difficult or complicated as it is made out to be. Meditation is simply putting yourself in a quiet, comfortable room and in a comfortable position so you could close your eyes and just relax your thoughts. If you feel that your thoughts are streaming uncontrollably, then just say to yourself, "that's OK" and then let them pass. You might want to concentrate on something rhythmic like your exhalation and inhalation or a phrase like "I am relaxed and still." There are many ways to relax, be still, and let your mind wander in any way it wants to go. That is meditation.

b. **Yoga:** This is another way to relax your thoughts by physically moving in various positions. You could practice yoga in the privacy of your home with some well-designed DVDs that guide you in various yoga poses and movements. Or you could attend a yoga center and participate in a class environment or have personal coaching with a yoga professional.

c. **Diaphragmatic breathing:** This is deep breathing in the diaphragm. The best way to do this is to put your hand over your belly button and, as you are breathing in, you want your belly to push your hand out as far as you can. You aren't trying to hold your stomach in; you want it to push out slowly and completely. Then when you begin to exhale, you want to think that you are trying to get your tummy right up to your spine as your hand moves in that direction as far as you can. Do this slowly. Repeat a number of times; it is very relaxing for you and your gut.

d. **Progressive muscle relaxation:** This will create total body relaxation. To set up for this technique, you probably will be ready to go to sleep, but you could do this anytime without getting ready to say goodnight. You want the room dark and cool. You also want to lie down on your back in bed and make yourself comfortable. You progressively will tighten groups of muscles and then relax them afterwards. Start with your feet. As you are lying in bed, squeeze and curl your toes and constrict your feet as tightly as you can. You probably will be holding your breath. Stay really tight, and then let go as you breath out. Then move to your legs, tightening and relaxing these muscles in the same way. Move up your body to your buttocks, abdomen, back, shoulders, neck, hands, arms, face, etc. Progressively tighten these muscles groups and then let go. After one round, your entire body will feel relaxed and stress-free. It has proved hugely beneficial for me. I actually learned the technique when I was in college many decades ago. At that time it was called Jacobsonian Relaxation.[222]

This list is far from exhaustive, but a great starting point. I have allowed my personal life to be affected by external stresses that I could have managed better if I only knew and practiced what I have described above. I have said it before, and I will continue to say it, "I am a work in progress."

So, where do you go from here? *You* need to make the choice: either be satisfied with this new information and do nothing with it, or be proactive and make some changes in your life. The next chapter gives you some clues on exactly how to get started.

20. All at Once--Or a Little at a Time?

You have read my philosophy for a healthier lifestyle in the last 19 chapters. If that made sense to you, getting started could mean not only a healthier mouth but also an overall healthier body. But where do you begin?

There are several ways to launch your new lifestyle journey. No matter which you eventually decide to do, it's critical that you understand this first:

Various macronutrients have been emphasized in the eating lifestyles of our primal ancestors, as well as modern-day hunter-gatherer societies. All these societies have survived and thrived. While it is important to include nutrient-dense whole foods in your diet, it is far more important to *avoid the foods that have been processed into acellular carbohydrates, unhealthy fats, and sugars*, along with the toxic substances that have been incorporated into most processed foods!

You could jump into the lifestyle I have described and make all the changes at once. Or, you could take various steps that lead to your goal, starting with some changes in your food choices. You might plan to progressively get involved over a few days, a few weeks, or even a more extended period of time.

Here is a progression to a healthier eating program, starting with a thirty-day challenge. Although some people may want to jump in all at once, there may be problems going too fast.

For example, research has shown that refined sugars may be as addictive as cocaine.[223] So, you could have intense cravings for refined carbohydrates during the first few weeks. It also would be reasonable to expect some withdrawal symptoms such as headaches, sluggishness, or a little "brain fog" after eliminating bad foods from your diet. But, you will get over these distressing symptoms in short order.

Others might have uncomfortable body reactions due to the sudden release of long-stored toxic substances. These reactions might manifest themselves in various ways such as acne, diarrhea, nausea, stomachaches, bloating, gas, muscle or joint aches, or headaches. For these reasons, some people prefer to take it slowly.

There are some people who may not have made up their minds that a new program is right for them. They might prefer to test the waters first.

Whichever way you decide to proceed, it will work for you if you are motivated to make it a success. It all starts in your head.

My personal story is a point in fact. I'm a person who jumps into something 100% if I believe in its benefits. When I went Primal in 2013, I did everything I have explained in the previous chapters as quickly as I could implement those changes for myself. During the first few weeks I had unbelievable cravings for my favorite carb--bagels. Before going Primal, I used to go to a well-known fast-food restaurant every Saturday for breakfast. It was the best multi-grain bagel with American cheese, a fried egg, and a crisp piece of salty fried chicken I had ever devoured.

Naturally, I couldn't eat only one; I needed to purchase two, which I gobbled up in a few minutes. After two, I was still hungry for another, but I couldn't be a pig. Once I started my primal eating lifestyle, I knew I had to give up the bagels, as well as all the other junk I had been consuming. It didn't take long for me to start *craving* those huge, delicious sandwiches. For the next three to four weeks, I could actually *taste* them in my mouth and feel them going down my throat. I yearned for them, but I was steadfast in my resolve not to give into the craving. Finally, after several weeks, the craving disappeared totally, and I haven't had a desire to eat one of those "death bombs" since. But, at the time, those cravings were both real *and* uncomfortable.

In order to control *your* cravings when you finally decide to take the leap, remember several things. First, you're not starting a new "diet." There is no hidden value here. What you see is what you get, because you're changing your lifestyle, one step at a time. Once you've changed over to a life of healthy eating, you'll remain there the rest of your life.

Of course, you *could* jump in a hundred percent from Day One. But regardless of how you choose to proceed, what matters most is that you do what you feel comfortable doing in your own time. Here is only one plan I follow for getting my own patients started.

First, I suggest a thirty-day challenge. Then, I propose you follow that up with a "Progressive Way to a Healthier Eating" program. After that, I analyze and summarize what foods are good and should be included in your lifestyle and what ones are bad and must be avoided. Finally, I discuss some general ideas on how to make things work for you.

Thirty-day challenge
Here is how my challenge to you works.

For the next thirty days (or whenever you want to start), stop eating all grains and products made from grains. The common grains include wheat, rye, barley, corn, rice, millet, and oats. Dump all foods that are made from these grains, such as cereals, breads made from wheat or other grain flours, pasta, crackers, cookies, cakes, muffins, bagels, pretzels, popcorn, rice biscuits, pancakes, pizza dough, and anything else whose ingredients label includes any grain product, no matter how much or how little.

Remember: grains irritate the lining of your gut, increase unhealthy bacteria in your gut that travel throughout your body, and interfere with your body's ability to absorb necessary nutrients from your foods. Grains can create inflammation in your body that may contribute to many chronic diseases. Grains can also produce irritations in your mouth, including ulcers and sores that never seem to heal.

I would also remove all pseudograins from your diet, even though they may be less troublesome than the cereal grains.

At the end of thirty days, you just might realize that you feel much better than you have felt for a long time. You may also discover that you have lost some of those pounds that you wanted to get rid of for a while. You even may decide to extend this experiment and include additional healthy choices to see what other positive outcomes you could enjoy.

After the thirty-day challenge, it's time you move on to my *Progressive Way to a Healthier Eating Program.*

Progressive way to a healthier eating program

Step 1: Eliminate unhealthy oils and fats

To begin my program, you'll need to eliminate unhealthy oils and fats from your diet. For the next fourteen days, remove all vegetable and seed oils, chemically produced trans fats, and partially hydrogenated fats. These oils and fats are toxic to your body. The only oil you'll want to put on your salads (in moderation) is macadamia, avocado, or extra virgin olive oil. When it comes to sautéing, the only fats you will use will be saturated fats such as coconut oil, butter or ghee from grass-fed cows, or other saturated fats (including tallow from grass-fed and grass-finished cattle or lard from pastured pigs).

Avoid *completely* all liquid polyunsaturated oils, such as canola oil, sunflower oil, safflower oil, corn oil, cottonseed oil, soybean oil, etc. If you are eating processed foods, you will need to investigate the ingredient lists of these foods to see if they contain any forbidden fats or oils.

Step 2: Eliminate all added sweeteners

For the next fourteen days, remove all added sugars and artificial sweeteners from your food intake. This includes all sodas and most can drinks. Refined and artificial sugars eventually stimulate your hormones to function poorly, creating cellular damage as well as damage to your gut lining and to your healthy gut bacteria. *Always look at* the labels on processed foods. Many are loaded with sugar and sugar aliases (high fructose corn syrup, agave nectar, cane juice, dextrose, etc.), even if the end product itself doesn't "taste" sweet. Artificial sweeteners consist of aspartame (NutraSweet®), sucralose (Splenda®), Saccharine, etc. If you absolutely must have a sweetener, use whole leaf stevia or local raw honey, a whole food--but do so sparingly.

Step 3: Eliminate all legumes

For the next fourteen days, remove all legumes from you diet. Legumes contain antinutrients that prevent certain minerals from being absorbed through your gut and damage the lining of the gut. Legumes include peanuts, black beans, garbanzo beans, pinto beans, lima beans, soybeans, lentils, etc.

Step 4: Eliminate pasteurized and homogenized milk products

Fourteen days later, remove all conventionally processed (that is, pasteurized and homogenized) milk products from your diet. Milk products have been physically, chemically, and biologically altered in such a way that it may be damaging to your gut lining and your hormone balance. Also, many people are lactose intolerant and/or sensitive to the casein protein in milk, which can mimic the gluten protein. Raw and non-homogenized milk and cheeses from cows, goats, and sheep are fine, as long as you can tolerate them.

Step 5: Eliminate most processed foods

Fourteen days after that, remove processed food products from your diet. These often contain chemical additives, preservatives, artificial ingredients, genetically modified foods, excessive unhealthy salt, unhealthy fats, refined sugars, acellular carbohydrates, and various other elements that may be toxic to your body over time. If the processed food has only healthy ingredients you recognize, you needn't be concerned. But if this food product has ingredients you cannot pronounce or offenders such as those above, avoid it.

In summary

Remember that there are bad and good food choices you can make, including these:

Bad food choices

- Vegetable oils (canola, safflower, sunflower, corn, soybean, etc.)
- Saturated fats from conventionally raised animals that are fed unnatural foods and given antibiotics, hormones, and other chemical agents
- Grains (wheat, rye, barley, oats, corn, rice, etc.) and grain products (breads, flour, cereals, popcorn, pizza dough, etc.)
- Products with artificial sweeteners or added sugars including all its aliases such as high-fructose corn syrup
- Legumes (soy, beans, lentils, peanuts, etc.)
- Pasteurized, ultra-pasteurized, and homogenized milk and milk products
- Processed foods that contain preservatives, hydrogenated fats, food coloring, added synthetic nutrients, and other harmful additives all of which may accumulate in your tissues.

Good food choices

- All products from animals (including their organs, such as liver, heart, kidney, brain, skin, and gelatinous parts) that have been pasture-raised or wild caught (ex. beef and buffalo that are grass-fed and grass-finished, seafood from fresh water or the ocean, free-range chickens and their eggs)
- Vegetables of various colors with an emphasis on non-starchy varieties and sea vegetables
- Fruits in moderation with an emphasis on deeply colored varieties, especially various berries and citrus
- Raw nuts and raw seeds in moderation after soaking to remove harmful elements.
- Probiotics (fermented foods such as sauerkraut, kimchi, possibly raw full-fat yogurt or possibly raw full-fat kefir), which will provide good bacteria to your body
- Prebiotics (examples: artichokes, asparagus, garlic, onions, resistant starch), to help feed the beneficial bacteria

- Organically grown foods, which have been shown to possess more essential nutrients than their non-organically grown counterparts
- Local produce (preferable to produce shipped in from hundreds of miles away)

I have included my favorite recipes at the end of the book so you can experiment with many exciting and new spices, seasonings, and textures, and, while doing so, actually retrain your taste buds.

Potentially tolerable food choices
- Raw dairy from pasture-raised goats or pasture-raised Guernsey cows (especially fermented raw dairy such as kefir and yogurt)
- Some legumes if soaked long enough and cooked long enough
- Fresh-ground organic coffee.

Sparingly-used food choices
- Dried fruits
- Raw honey
- White potatoes
- White rice

Additional tips for success

1. To generate health, you need to remove the bad (such as toxic substances, stress, and poor food choices) and add the good (such as whole fresh food, sleep, exercise, and the great outdoors). Food will be medicine. You will eat nutrient-dense foods, and your cells will self-correct. Let's get the ball rolling! Here are some tips.
   - Try to get your family on the same page as you. Mutual support makes a change of lifestyle easier over the long haul.

- Identify the real reason you want to make a change in your life.
- Set a specific *start* date.
- Remove the unhealthy foods from your kitchen (so that you will eliminate any temptations), and stock it with the foods, herbs, and spices that create health.
- Learn how to navigate your supermarket to purchase the healthy foods and how to read the "ingredient list" and "nutrition facts" on food labels.
- Consider joining a CSA[224] (Community-Supported Agriculture) to get local, fresh, organic produce weekly.
- Develop simple cooking skills to prepare these delicious and healthy foods, purchase the kitchen items you need, and check out some whole-food cookbooks in the Appendix of this book.
- Consider purchasing a high performance blender such as the Vitamix®[225] or NutriBullet Rx®[226], which will make it very easy to "eat" your leafy greens in the form of a smoothie anytime and anywhere.
- Stop all nicotine use. *PERIOD!*
- If you have intestinal problems, you may want to consider stopping all caffeine, alcohol, and any other substances that could be interfering with your health. (Appropriate amounts of caffeine and alcohol may be added back later.)
- Be aware that you get most of your vitamin D from the sun and *not* from your diet. If necessary, rely upon a whole-food supplement that can assist your intake of vitamin D as I discussed in *Give Yourself Nutrient-Dense Nourishment* in the previous chapter.
- Since blood sugar levels are a significant predictor of potential future degenerative diseases, you

should invest in a Blood Glucose Monitor. Frequent testing is not only for diabetics!

2. As you begin to make healthy food choices, your carbohydrate cravings will disappear and your digestive hormones will become balanced. Probably the most important thing to wrap your head around is simply that hormones control many aspects of our lives. Most aspects of this healthy eating style are designed to drive lifestyle changes that will keep hormones at levels necessary for natural balance. As your hormones become balanced, they will tell your body when you need to eat and when you are satiated.

3. You should eat when you are hungry. Some people may want to eat more food during the first meal of the day and then taper off in quantity as the day progresses. These are individual preferences. It would be best not to eat within three hours of going to bed. Sometimes, eating closer to bedtime may help you sleep better as I described in getting restorative sleep. Many people will eat three meals a day spaced out about every five hours. However, current research suggests that skipping a meal especially if you are not hungry has been shown to assist with healthy metabolism. This is called *intermittent fasting*.

4. At each meal, try to create the Perfect Plate, ideally consisting of half or more of non-starchy vegetables with healthy fats, one-quarter of some type of protein with all of its healthy fats, and one-quarter of whole food fats (such as avocados or nuts). You may also include a small portion of a starchy vegetable (such as a sweet potato) or possibly a small portion of berries or citrus fruits.

5. If you're trying to lose weight, eating less fruits and starches will accelerate your weight loss. This healthy eating program is not about calories; it is about quality of food. One hundred calories of a chocolate cookie are not the same as 100 calories of broccoli. A fact that was

uncovered from the Human Genome Project was that *food is information,* that controls your gene expression, hormones, and metabolism.[227,228]

6. If you cannot measure it, you cannot improve it. - Lord Kelvin

   Taking measurements will help keep track of your progress and will help guide you to make necessary changes. Waist size, hip size, blood pressure, and percentage of body fat are measurements that will change as your body becomes healthier. Taking your fasting blood sugar with a Blood Glucose Monitor will show you how well you are controlling your blood sugar. Photographs will be your visual testimonials. Have a close friend or spouse take a picture of you in your bathing suit before you start and then once a month thereafter. You will see the unfolding changes. Although you might be most concerned about your weight, weight is the *least* important measurement.

7. When traveling or in an emergency, putting together a handy *Emergency Food Pack* such as this one may prove handy.
   - Plastic bag of raw almonds, cashews, walnuts, pecans, or macadamia nuts
   - Plastic bag of celery or cucumbers
   - Plastic bag of homemade kale chips (see Appendix)
   - Can or plastic bag of wild salmon with bones and skin
   - Can or plastic bag of sardines with bones and skin
   - Healthy whole-food protein bar (ex: AMRAP Refuel Bars®[229], but be aware that these bars do contain raw honey, and they must be used sparingly!)
   - Bottle of water
   - Spoon/Fork/Napkins

8. In addition to the healthy eating lifestyle I have emphasized, you should implement at your own pace the various areas I discussed in the section, *Master Methods of*

Maintenance. Start brushing your teeth with coconut oil and baking soda. Take more walks. Get outside in the sun a few more days of the week. Start incorporating a more efficient exercise program. Try standing as much as you can as opposed to sitting. Go to sleep at a time that will allow your body to get the hours it needs to restore itself. Experiment with some methods to reduce the stress in your life. Take little steps to reform who you are and what you do.

21. Modifying the *Lifestyle-Repair Plan* for Specific Concerns

Think of the *Lifestyle-Repair Plan* we explored in Chapter 19 as the foundation for your new lifestyle. It's designed to decrease chronic inflammation, which is the precursor to so many diseases. Incorporating the *Plan's* nutrient-dense diet and lifestyle changes will enhance your body's ability to be strong and function as it was designed. But, there are some modifications that can be considered for specific health disorders or concerns. *Note:* Be sure to check with your medical doctor to see if these modifications could work for you. Everyone is an individual with individual differences and needs. What works for one may not work for another.

The following Baker's Dozen conditions come from a little "fine tuning" of the *Plan*. If any pertain to you, allow at least two months of tweaking before expecting to see a change in your circumstances. Many of these modifications are repeated for several of the listed issues:

Periodontal Disease

Dietary modifications that may improve your overall mouth health include these:

- Limit the carbohydrate density of your foods to less than 23%. (See the section on Carbohydrate Density in the beginning of this book.)
- Consider brushing with local, raw honey. I described some of the benefits of local, raw honey in the section, *G: Give yourself nutrient-dense nourishment.*
- Maintain a healthy gut microbiome by eating fermented *every day!*
- Feed the healthy gut bacteria daily with soluble fiber foods such as dark-colored fruits, non-starchy vegetables, starchy tubers such as sweet potatoes, and resistant starch. (See the subsection of *Prebiotics* under *Supplements* in *G: Give yourself nutrient-dense nourishment.*)
- Obtain necessary micronutrients from seaweeds.

- Eat oily fish such as salmon, sardines, and anchovies to get healthy levels of DHA as well as Vitamin D.
- Be sure to get bioavailable levels of calcium from bones and bone broth, dark leafy greens, canned salmon with bones, and raw grass-fed dairy products (assuming you can tolerate the lactose).
- Magnesium is an important micronutrient that is naturally available in such foods as Swiss chard, spinach, pumpkin seeds, Brazil nuts, and raw cocoa.
- Another important micronutrient is Vitamin C, which is readily available in such foods as broccoli and citrus.
- Eat liver and egg yolks from pastured chickens and ghee from grass-fed cows to obtain Vitamin K2 (which is critical for proper function of Vitamins A and D, as well as for calcium metabolism). Hard cheese from grass-fed cows is also high in Vitamin K2.
- Practice excellent oral hygiene methods.
- Be sure to obtain healthy levels of Vitamin D from the sun, your diet, and/or proper supplements. One of my suggestions under *Supplements* in *G: Give yourself nutrient-dense nourishment* is Butter Oil/Fermented Cod Liver Oil from GreenPasture®. (The blood test I described earlier is the only way to know what your levels are.)

Weight Loss

When you are eating according to the *Plan*, your hormones tend to balance out. Your body will tell you when you are hungry and when you have had enough to eat. However, when your weight is the issue in the beginning of your health journey, specific modifications might help you achieve your desired weight.

- Emphasize reducing the carbohydrate load in your meals. Do this by *increasing* the amount of protein you eat to help satisfy your hunger. In addition, increase the amount of non-starchy vegetables on your plate while reducing the amount of starchy vegetables. The greatest amount of carbs will come from the sugars in fruit, so reduce the amount of fruit you eat. If you are eating some fruit, favor the less caloric ones, such as the various berries (blueberries, raspberries, blackberries, strawberries, etc.).

- Avoid snacking.
- While healthy fats are satiating and delicious, eating them in abundance while trying to lose weight could become a problem since they are high in calories. Continue to use healthy fats such as ghee, coconut oil, olive oil, and fats from pastured animals, but do so in moderation. Reducing the quantity of healthy fats is a good thing until you have reached your goal of weight loss.
- Avoid dairy products with the exception of a small amount of butter or ghee since dairy products have been implicated in weight gain for some people.
- Try to eat within an eight-hour window, which is called intermittent fasting as I have discussed in the *M: Master Methods of Maintenance.* For example, I usually finish my dinner between seven and 8 p.m., and I don't eat anything after that until the next day at about noon. Essentially, my body is fasting from 8 p.m. until noon, or roughly 16 hours. That leaves me an eight-hour eating window from noon to 8 p.m.
- Support your gut health by eating foods that feed your gut microbiome (examples: fermented foods such as sauerkraut, kombucha, yogurt, and kefir plus various probiotic supplement preparations to add to your gut flora when necessary).
- Include daily non-exercise movement such as walking about 10,000 steps a day if you can. Use a pedometer to keep track until you get an idea of what it takes in your routine to accomplish this.
- Stand as much as you can instead of sitting. I personally use a stand-up desk at home when I am using my computer.

- Create an efficient exercise program that incorporates high intensity interval training once or twice a week as well as moderate aerobic exercise two to three days a week.
- Allow seven to eight hours a night for restorative sleep in a room that is cool, dark, and quiet.
- Reduce your total stress load levels.

High Cholesterol and Heart Disease

Before discussing the modifications to diet and lifestyle, here is what science has to say about cholesterol and heart disease.

Our liver makes about 75% of our cholesterol; about 25% comes from our diet. When total cholesterol intake goes down, the body makes more; when intake goes up, the body makes less.

Cholesterol is essential for life, making up a significant part of cell membranes, which are essential for the cell to function. In addition to cholesterol making up about half of a cell's membrane, it is also the precursor to sex hormones, adrenal hormones, and other hormones of the body. The myelin sheath that protects neurons is 20% cholesterol. Cholesterol helps the intestinal wall to stay intact, and it functions as an antioxidant to prevent oxidative damage from free radicals.

Cholesterol is fat-soluble. Since our blood is mostly water, cholesterol cannot be dissolved in the blood alone. Cholesterol must be combined to special proteins (called *apolipoproteins*) that are bound to fats, which are then called *lipoproteins*. Lipoproteins are categorized by their density. Examples are low-density lipoproteins (LDL) and high-density lipoproteins (HDL).

When your doctor orders a blood test, it usually checks your cholesterol levels. This test actually measures the amount of cholesterol that the lipoproteins contain.

Lipoproteins are essential to the human body. They transport cholesterol to and from tissues and eventually back to the liver to be processed and excreted. Lipoproteins are also the transport vehicles for fat-soluble vitamins A, D, E, and K and various antioxidants.

An important factor in heart disease is the actual number of LDL particles flowing through the coronary arteries. When a large number of LDL particles exists, the sheer number forces some of them to leave the blood and penetrate the cell-layer-thick lining of the artery, thereby entering the artery wall.

Therefore, the driving factor for plaque formation in the arterial wall is not the amount of cholesterol in the lipoprotein but rather the number of lipoprotein particles flowing in the blood.

Your total cholesterol, total LDL-cholesterol, and total HDL-cholesterol levels are not as important as the total number of LDL particles.

Another important factor in heart disease is the oxidation of LDL particles. Oxidation is similar to a cut apple turning brown or steel rusting. When our body's normal antioxidant systems are weakened, oxidation can occur in the LDL particles. Oxidation produces free radicals, which are damaging to cells and DNA.

Oxidized LDL particles can initiate atherosclerosis or hardening of the arteries. Oxidized LDL particles are denser than non-oxidized LDL particles and are most damaging to the lining of the arteries. When these oxidized LDL particles embed into the artery wall, they can cause collagen to form that can eventually rupture and create heart attacks.

So, what causes an increase in the number of LDL particles, and what causes them to become oxidized? These answers will go a long way to understanding how to reduce the risk of cardiovascular disease.

The main causes for an increase in the number of LDL particles are the presence of the risk factors of metabolic syndrome (i.e. high triglycerides, low HDL, and insulin and leptin resistance) plus various genetic factors. Other causes include poor thyroid function, iodine deficiency, and viral and bacterial infections.

The main causes for oxidative damage to the LDL particles are the type of fats that make up the structure of the LDL particles, the level of antioxidants incorporated in the LDL particles, and the degree of oxidative stress present. Omega-6 fatty acids especially from vegetable oils are inflammatory and can oxidize rapidly. If these fats are abundant in the LDL particles, they could contribute to the oxidation of LDL particles.

If the original production of LDL in the liver does not incorporate enough antioxidants into the LDL particles, then these LDL particles could become oxidized faster. Similarly, the oxidative stress load could become excessive from smoking, chronic stress, environmental toxic substances, infections, physical inactivity, and iron overload.

Diet modifications to decrease overall risk

- Replace carbohydrates with saturated fats in your meals to reduce the level of triglycerides, thereby decreasing the number of LDL particles. (Example: instead of eating sweet potatoes and high-glycemic fruits such as bananas with a meal, replace them with non-starchy leafy greens sautéed in coconut oil or ghee.) Note that there are some people who may be overly sensitive to saturated fats, which may need to be reduced.
- Consider eating local, raw honey as I described in the section, *G: Give yourself nutrient-dense nourishment*.
- Eliminate snacks.
- Practice intermittent fasting.
- Increase fatty fish and shellfish such as salmon, mackerel, herring, sardines, anchovies, oysters, mussels, or fish eggs to increase healthy omega-3 fatty acids as well as many other nutrients.
- Increase monosaturated fats such as olives, olive oil, macadamia nuts, and avocados.
- Increase antioxidant foods as found in a rainbow of colors of fruits (such as berries) and vegetables, organ and red meats, and eggs.

- Increase polyphenol-rich foods as found in green tea, dark-colored fruits and vegetables, dark chocolate, coffee, turmeric, and herbs and spices.
- Moderately increase tree nuts such as almonds, Brazil nuts, cashews, walnuts, and pistachios but be careful with the quantity you consume, since nuts are high in omega-6 fatty acids.
- Increase fermented foods such as sauerkraut, kimchi, kombucha, and raw yogurt or raw kefir (if you can tolerate lactose).
- Increase soluble fibers such as dandelion greens, onions, garlic, and asparagus.

Lifestyle modifications to decrease overall risk
- Decrease levels of stress.
- Increase restorative sleep.
- Increase efficient exercise.

High Blood Pressure
Medication may be necessary because chronic high blood pressure could be life threatening. However, changes in diet and lifestyle could reduce levels of high blood pressure to the point where you can reduce or eliminate such medications entirely.

Immediate dietary modifications
- Eliminate all refined sugar.
- Increase potassium in your diet from sweet potatoes, plantains, bananas, canned tomatoes avocados, and salmon.
- Increase DHA-containing animal foods such as salmon, herring, sardines, anchovies, oysters, and mussels.
- Increase magnesium consumption from such foods as nuts, seeds, spinach, and beet greens.
- Increase daily consumption of >80% dark chocolate or 100% organic raw cacao.
- Drink two to three cups of hibiscus tea daily. (Research suggests hibiscus tea has diuretic properties, dilates

arteries, and inhibits the release of hormones that constrict blood vessels.)

- Include seaweed such as wakame and kelp in soups.

Lifestyle modifications

- Get plenty of restorative sleep.
- Exercise more.
- Try Stress reduction, including meditation and deep breathing.
- Get out in the sun. The UV light from the sun stimulates nitric oxide in the body, which in turn dilates blood vessels, reducing blood pressure.

Digestive Problems

Digestive diseases run the gamut, causing episodes of diarrhea, constipation, pain, and gas. Some named diseases include GERD (Gastroesophageal Reflux Disease), irritable bowel syndrome (IBS), and inflammatory bowel diseases (IBD), which includes Crohn's disease and ulcerative colitis. All of these may have similar underlying factors such as:

- Overgrowth of bacteria in the small intestine, called SIBO (small intestinal bacterial overgrowth)
- Dysbiosis, which is an imbalance of bad bacteria over good bacteria
- Intestinal permeability (leaky gut) where openings in the one-cell-layer-thick gut lining are breaking down and allowing unwanted material to flow or leak into the blood system
- Chronic infections involving bacteria, parasites, and yeast
- Breakdown in the gut/brain communication system
- Gut disorders that contribute to various other functions of the body, including immune system malfunction; thyroid gland malfunction; and adrenal gland malfunction, since chronic systemic inflammation affects cortisol production.

Diet modifications

- Reduce foods that are in the class of FODMAPs (fermentable *oligosaccharides, disaccharides, monosaccharides,* and *polyols*). These are carbohydrates that cannot be absorbed well and are easily fermented by gut bacteria. They can cause water to be drawn into the large intestine, resulting in gas, pain, and diarrhea. There is a large list of foods that fit this category. The major sugars included are fructose, fructan, lactose, galactose, and polyols (sugar alcohols).
- Reduce foods with insoluble fiber because these fibers are irritating to the intestines (examples: Beet root, parsnips, apples, raspberries, spinach, turnips, and okra).
- Increase fermented foods such as sauerkraut and kimchi.
- Drink or eat one to two cups of homemade bone broth daily.
- Increase soluble fiber from fruits and starchy veggies such as sweet potatoes, plantains, yucca, and taro. (Individuals with GERD and IBD may need to limit these foods.)
- Decrease alcohol usage.
- Note: In the early treatment of digestive disease, the diet could be very restrictive. However, as the gut heals, many of the restricted foods could be reintroduced.

Lifestyle modifications

- Decrease stress
- Increase restorative sleep
- Participate in efficient exercise

Blood Sugar Disorders

High- and low-blood sugar diseases are metabolic disorders that are usually related to lifestyle. Contributing factors include acellular carbohydrate consumption, lack of exercise and non-exercise movement, chronic stress, inadequate sleep, digestive diseases, and environmental toxic substances.

Diet modifications

- Increase protein to stabilize high and low blood sugar levels.
- Eat fermented foods such as sauerkraut, kimchi, and kombucha to support good gut bacteria.
- Eat fermentable fibers such as fruits and both starchy and non-starchy vegetables to feed good gut bacteria.
- Include three to four tablespoons of resistant starch (unmodified organic potato starch) dissolved in a glass of water daily to feed good gut bacteria. But, start off with only 1 teaspoon per day, and work up to the required dose.
- If sugar is too high: avoid snacks and consider intermittent fasting.
- If sugar is too low: eat every two to three hours starting with a protein breakfast.

Lifestyle modifications

- Get more exercise.
- Get enough restorative sleep.
- Eliminate stress from your life.

Anxiety, Depression, and Cognitive Disorders

Brain disorders have been shown to have three distinct common precursors: decreased quality of nutrient-dense foods, intestinal permeability and *dysbiosis,* and chronic systemic inflammation.

Diet modifications

- Reduce the quantity of FODMAP foods in the diet because they encourage digestive disorders as discussed in the modifications for Digestive Disorders.
- Increase glycine-rich foods. Glycine is an amino acid that supports the production of serotonin. Foods high in glycine are the gelatinous cuts of meat such as oxtail, brisket, and chuck roast. Other foods high in glycine are homemade bone broth and egg yolks.

- Increase the consumption of fermented foods because they improve the gut microbiome, which in turn supports brain health.
- Research the GAPS (Gut And Psychology Syndrome) Diet. Created by Natasha Campbell-McBride, MD, it has been shown to help many people with these disorders. Here is a website to gain further information[230].

Lifestyle modifications
- Efficient exercise is critical.
- Restorative sleep is critical.
- Stress management is critical.
- In addition, sunlight exposure is important.

Thyroid Disorders

All cells in the body have receptors for thyroid hormones. Therefore, all bodily functions require thyroid hormones to function efficiently.

Hypothyroidism (a *decrease* in thyroid hormones) is more common than hyperthyroidism (an *increase* in thyroid hormones). Hyperthyroidism is also more serious than hypothyroidism since it is associated with an increased risk of heart attack, stroke, and death.

A large percentage of thyroid disorders are autoimmune. The most common form of autoimmune *hypothyroid* disorder is called Hasimotto's Disease where the body's immune system attacks the normal thyroid gland progressively destroying its ability to produce thyroid hormone. The most common form of *hyperthyroid* disorder is called Graves' Disease where the thyroid gland becomes enlarged and overactive. Since diet and lifestyle efficiency are important for the immune system, regulating them may be the first concern in treating thyroid disorders.

Another major cause of thyroid disorders is iodine and/or selenium deficiencies. These two minerals are essential for thyroid hormone production. Iodine is part of the structure of thyroid hormones, and a deficiency of iodine can cause hypothyroidism as well as swelling of the thyroid gland, which is called goiter. (Also, an excess of iodine may cause goiter or exacerbate autoimmune thyroid disorders.) Selenium affects the conversion of T4 (the inactive form of thyroid hormone) into T3 (the active form of thyroid hormone).

Diet modifications

- Limit goitrogenic foods. *Goitrogens* are substances that interfere with iodine uptake in the thyroid. In small amounts, these foods may increase the need for iodine. In large amounts, they may damage the thyroid gland. Steaming or boiling goitrogenic foods may decrease their damaging qualities; so, consuming cooked goitrogens is better than consuming them raw. Goitrogen foods consist of gluten, soy, broccoli, peanuts, strawberries, kale, and other vegetables.
- Eat foods that contain biologically available selenium and iodine.
- Reduce foods that can trigger an immune response. (See the Autoimmune section in this chapter.)
- Avoid very low carbohydrate consumption and very low protein consumption. Adequate amounts of carbs and protein are necessary to promote the release of insulin, which in turn is necessary for the conversion of T4 into T3.
- If you have gut disorders, gut health must be restored. (See Gut Disorders in this chapter.)

Lifestyle modifications

- Manage stress.
- Get some sun because the ultraviolet light in the form of UVA and UVB can help reduce the effects of an overactive immune system.

Autoimmune Disorders

Autoimmune disorders occur when the body's normal defense mechanisms begin to attack healthy cells. The list of diseases that are or may be autoimmune is staggering. Here is a partial list of some common diseases considered to be autoimmune:

- Addison's Disease: adrenal hormone insufficiency
- Celiac Disease: a reaction to gluten (found predominantly in wheat, rye, and barley) that causes damage to the lining of the small intestine
- Graves' Disease: overactive thyroid gland
- Hashimoto's Disease: inflammation of the thyroid gland
- Inflammatory Bowel Disease: a group of inflammatory diseases of the colon and small intestine
- Pernicious Anemia: decrease in red blood cells caused by inability to absorb vitamin B-12
- Psoriasis: a skin condition that causes redness and irritation as well as thick, flaky, silver-white patches
- Reactive Arthritis: inflammation of joints, urethra, and eyes; may cause sores on the skin and mucus membranes
- Rheumatoid Arthritis: inflammation of joints and surrounding tissues
- Scleroderma: a connective tissue disease that causes changes in skin, blood vessels, muscles, and internal organs
- Sjögren's Syndrome: destroys the glands that produce tears and saliva causing dry eyes and mouth; may affect kidneys and lungs
- Systemic Lupus Erythematosus: affects skin, joints, kidneys, brain, and other organs
- Type 1 Diabetes: destruction of insulin producing cells in the pancreas
- Vitiligo: white patches on the skin caused by loss of pigment

Autoimmune diseases in particular occur most often when these three elements are present:

- A genetic predisposition for a particular disease
- An environmental trigger such as toxic substances, specific foods, infections and gut dysbiosis

- Damage to the gut lining (leaky gut)

Treatment for autoimmune diseases must start with the removal of all triggers and the repairing of the gut. Improvements in diet and lifestyle are foundational for healing.

Diet modifications:

Remove the following trigger foods (some but not all may be the offenders):

- Eggs
- Foods that are members of the Nightshade family (including potatoes, tomatoes, sweet and hot peppers, eggplant, tomatillos, pepinos, pimentos, paprika, cayenne but not black pepper)
- Dairy

Add or *increase* foods that support the production of glutathione, which is the master antioxidant of the body:

- Collagen-rich animal parts, such as bone and cartilage, because they contain glycine, which is an amino acid that is required in glutathione synthesis (foods such as homemade bone broth and gelatinous cuts of meat including skin, chuck roast, and oxtail)
- Polyphenol-rich fruits and vegetables, such as berries, peaches, pears, pomegranates, purple sweet potatoes, broccoli, garlic, cabbage, and spinach
- Selenium-rich foods, such as Brazil nuts, ocean fish, and poultry
- EPA and DHA foods, which have omega-3 fatty acids that are anti-inflammatory (foods such as salmon, mackerel, herring, sardines, and anchovies)
- Vitamin D foods, such as high-vitamin cod liver oil, fatty fish (salmon, mackerel, herring, sardines, and anchovies), pastured duck, and pastured chicken eggs
- Organ meats, herbs and spices, nuts and seeds, cocoa, seaweed (because of its many micronutrients)
- Fermented foods that support a healthy gut microbiome

Lifestyle modifications

- Reduce chronic stress from all stressors
- Improve sleep
- Exercise efficiently
- Get sun to benefit from ultraviolet light that improves the immune system

Adrenal Fatigue Syndrome

Adrenal fatigue syndrome involves the hypothalamus-pituitary-adrenal (HPA) axis. The HPA axis controls our response to stress. Cortisol, a hormone produced in the adrenal cortex, is the primary hormone that regulates our stress response. Practically all of our organ systems are affected by stress and cortisol. If you are experiencing adrenal fatigue, then dietary and lifestyle changes will be necessary.

Dietary modifications

- Eat carbohydrates in moderation (not too high and not too low). You will need to experiment to determine the amount of carbs per day that works best for you.
- Eat a high-protein breakfast because it helps regulate blood sugar.
- If you have low blood sugar, your adrenals will produce cortisol to elevate your sugar level. This can stress the adrenal gland. Eating every two to three hours can stabilize your blood sugar levels and reduce the overproduction of cortisol.
- If your blood pressure is low, decrease excess potassium foods because potassium can decrease your blood pressure. You should consume these in moderation: bananas, dried figs, raisins, dates, potatoes, and sweet potatoes. (Monitor your blood pressure at home.)
- If your blood pressure is low, increase sea salt consumption to taste. Sodium will increase aldosterone hormone, which

is produced in the adrenal gland and may be low in adrenal fatigue. (Monitor your blood pressure at home.)

- Avoid caffeine and alcohol until your adrenals recover because they will stress the adrenal gland.

Lifestyle modifications

- Reduce all stress.
- Sleep restoratively and rest during the day as necessary.
- Exercise efficiently, but eliminate *excessive* exercise.
- Get outdoors and enjoy nature and the sun.

Acne, Eczema, Psoriasis, and Other Skin Conditions

Our skin is influenced by other organ systems. Anxiety, depression, stress, and the gut microbiome play huge roles in the health of the skin. Heal the gut and chronic inflammation may subside along with numerous other degenerative diseases. The first effort to healthier skin is the eating and lifestyle program in my *Plan*. Especially healthy for skin are the organ meats and bone broth.

However, some people with skin disorders have an intolerance to a natural chemical in the body called histamine. Among other purposes, histamine is also a mediator of the symptoms of an allergic reaction (redness, swelling, itching, hives, red eyes, nasal congestion, runny nose, headaches, and skin rashes). Histamine intolerance can occur if the body does not break down histamine properly or if the gut microbiome is allowing more histamine-producing bacteria to proliferate. Histamine intolerance is not a sudden condition; it builds slowly over time until symptoms occur clinically.

Dietary modifications may help with SOME skin conditions. Not everyone will need to eliminate all of these, and those that are eliminated could be reintroduced as symptoms subside. Do give thought to eliminating these foods if your skin conditions have not improved after being on the *Plan* for at least three months:

- Seafood
- Eggs

- Processed meats such as bacon, sausage, salami, and peperoni
- Fermented foods
- Citrus fruits
- Berries
- Dried fruit
- Spinach
- Tomatoes
- Many spices
- Tea, alcohol, chocolate, cocoa
- Vinegar and products containing vinegar

Another food group that could be exacerbating skin conditions could be the foods in the FODMAP group. If reducing the histamine-containing foods has not improved your skin conditions, try reducing or eliminating the foods in the FODMAP group.

Lifestyle modifications
- UV light has been shown to help some skin conditions. Sun exposure for ten to fifteen minutes a day, two to three days a week may be beneficial.
- Get restorative sleep. Sleep deprivation can cause increased systemic inflammation and disruption of hormones that could lead to skin disorders.
- Get efficient exercise. Exercise will decrease systemic inflammation, increase blood flow, and decrease stress. If you have adrenal fatigue, then your exercise program should be gentle.
- Use stress reduction techniques I have previously discussed. Stress is a major player in disrupting the gut microbiome and affecting the immune system.

Fertility, Pregnancy, and Breastfeeding
Research has shown that the mother's nutritional status leading up to and during pregnancy affects her baby's health. This is true not

only at birth and during early childhood, but also continuing throughout adult life.

The anti-inflammatory, nutrient-dense diet that makes up the eating style of my *Plan* is the foundation diet for women wishing to conceive and who are pregnant. However, there are *superfoods* listed below that *enhance* the nutritional quality of her diet for fertility, pregnancy, and breastfeeding. Moms can modify their diets by increasing consumption of these seven nutrient-dense foods:

- Liver, the most nutrient-dense food on the planet
- Egg yolks, which have been called "nature's multivitamin"
- Fatty fish, such as salmon, mackerel, herring, and sardines, all high in DHA and EPA
- Cod liver oil, which is high in Vitamins A and D as well as EPA and DHA
- Grass-fed, raw dairy, which is rich in saturated fats, CLA (conjugated linoleic acid), and fat soluble vitamins A, D, K2, and E (if Mom can tolerate lactose)
- Fermented foods, which help support a healthy gut microbiome
- Homemade bone broth, which supplies nutrients to support gut health as well as overall health

Asthma

A specific diet has not been shown to eliminate the symptoms of asthma. However, for some asthmatics, the elimination of gluten has reduced or eliminated the effects of their previous asthma triggers. Since my *Lifestyle-Repair Plan* is an anti-inflammatory way of eating, many people have noticed improvements in their asthma episodes by eating this way. Modifying the Plan in these ways may prove to be beneficial for asthmatics:

- Increase vitamin D and omega-3 fatty acids. Eating fatty fish such as salmon, herring, mackerel, sardines and anchovies are good sources as well as cod liver oil. The best source of Vitamin D is the sun as I have described previously.

- Increase fruits and vegetables, which are good sources of antioxidants.
- Reduce sulfite-containing foods, which can trigger asthma symptoms in some people. Sulfites can be found in wine, dried fruits, pickles, and fresh and frozen shrimp.
- Maintain a healthy weight since being overweight can worsen asthma.
- New research has shown that enhancing the microbiome in newborn babies may reduce the risk of asthma.

22. Can I Cheat?

I hope you haven't gotten to this point only to think about how you could cheat your way through it all. Removing unhealthy food choices and replacing them with healthy ones is a lifestyle change. It's not a fad diet that comes to an end allowing you to return to old eating habits. As a matter of fact, if you eliminated only the acellular carbs and foods that have a high carbohydrate density, you would have greatly reduced your food cravings, and your body would be healthier--your mouth, much better for the experience. Your desire to cheat should have decreased. Nonetheless, to answer the question, "Can I cheat?"

"Yes, you can."

Of course, you need to define what *cheating* means.

As Mark Sisson[231] and Dr. Loren Cordain[232] have stated in their writings, the 80/20-rule or the 85/15-rule work. That means, if you are eating the foods that are part of the nutrient-dense lifestyle 80-85% of the time, then 15-20% of the time you could go off track and still be okay. That *off-track* time would be considered *cheating* or maybe just *indulging off the grid.*

I am motivated, perhaps beyond most people's understanding. You might have calculated that I am almost 70 years old as I write this. At this point in my lifestyle change, which only began in 2013, I am a fat burner. That means that I usually consume less than 150 grams of carbohydrates a day (without actually counting grams but by making healthier food choices), and for the most part I have no carb cravings. I can effectively burn stored fat for energy throughout the day. In addition, I generally skip a formal breakfast because I am not hungry and start my first meal after the noon hour and end my last meal of the day by 8 p.m. (intermittent fasting). But, most people are not like me. I definitely get that.

Interestingly, there may be some actual benefits to *cheating* or *indulging off the grid.*

Break the monotony

For some people, staying the course of eating healthy can be difficult. Sometimes that burger with all the drippings, condiments, and perfect bun sounds awesome. Other times your buddies and you are out and about, and a pizza with a beer would top off a perfect evening. So, you join them by *indulging off the grid*. That's okay. It's a break from what may appear to you to be the *monotony of sticking to a strict food regimen*. There is even a study that demonstrates how occasional overindulging can improve your results.[233] Just don't do it often. Of course, that's not true for everyone. For those with autoimmune diseases, allergic reactions, and damaged guts, even an occasional *indulgence* could cause unpleasant and serious reactions.

The hormesis effect

Hormesis is the term for generally favorable biological responses to low exposures to toxic substances and other stressors. That's why plants build up phytonutrients in their cell structure to ward off potential pests and disease. The stress created externally will build strength internally. Just as the plant becomes stronger and more resistant, the human body can become stronger and more resistant. Some research has demonstrated that eating some bad foods at times might improve overall health.[234, 235, 236] But, again, don't make this a routine excuse because of some research to *indulge off the grid*.

Kick-start your metabolism

If you had reduced your carbohydrate intake significantly and for a prolonged time, you actually could have depressed your metabolic rate[237] and stalled your weight loss[238]. When you eat a big meal especially high in carbohydrates, you could trigger specific hormones to restart your weight loss goals.

If you have been motivated to make a lifestyle change as I have described throughout this book, then you are most likely not thinking about actively cheating. You may occasionally want to eat foods that do not have the ideal nutrient density that you would otherwise eat, and that's okay. You may go out with the guys or gals and decide you will indulge in a way that you normally would not do, and that's okay, too. These are the exceptions and certainly not the rule. I can go to almost any restaurant, even fast-food types, and find something on the menu that I will eat. The important thing for me is this: I know what I *won't* eat, and everything else is just fine.

Think about where you are mentally now compared to where you were when you started reading this book. I am a perfect example of a person who has embraced a new lifestyle that has changed my life. How could I ever consider going back to the way I was when I know that this Primal lifestyle has saved my life?

Best of luck pursuing your new life.

23. Myth vs. Reality

There is much evidence-based research today that has created a path for the discerning person to follow to regain and maintain the health that the human body was designed to possess. I have known people who were able to accept that revelation, and I've known people who weren't. Which one are you? If you're the former, then the path for you starts with you making a decision to change your life--to change your health.

Some people need a personal tipping point such as a stroke or a heart attack to make a change. Some people need a love-of-their-life addition, such as the birth of a granddaughter or a grandson to institute a change. Some people are motivated after they get a new job or move into a new home. Some people only need information that they never knew existed. Which discerning person are you?

Here are some statements that used to be considered *facts* by the scientific community but have since been determined to be incorrect. My responses are in the form of *Consider This*:

"Fat makes you fat."

Consider This: Carbohydrates make you fat because of excessive insulin production. Healthy fats satisfy your hunger and provide fuel. Generally, ingested fat will not become storage fat unless insulin is excessive from too many carbs, or you are too sedentary.

"Running 5 miles a day is good heart exercise."

Consider This: Chronic exercise produces oxidative stress, is unhealthy for the cardiovascular system, and discourages fat burning. Lifting heavy things a couple of times a week and sprinting once a week are much healthier for your heart as well as your waistline and need only take ten to twenty minutes each. In addition, a couple of hours of aerobic exercise spaced out during the week and physical non-exercise movement throughout each day will round out a healthy routine.

"Breakfast is the healthiest meal of the day."

Consider This: The most important time to eat is when you are hungry. If your hormones are in balance, you may actually not need to eat until noon or later. When you do eat, each meal conceptually should be a plate of food partitioned like this: at least half of the plate should include non-starchy veggies either raw or sautéed in healthy fat; a quarter of the plate should be some type of free-range or wild-caught protein including their natural fats; and the last quarter could be made up of some of these--some nuts or seeds, deeply colored fruit (such as berries or citrus), and a small starchy vegetable.

"Whole grains have plenty of nutrients."

Consider This: Grains contain elements that irritate the gut and interfere with normal absorption of necessary minerals. Grains were introduced into the human diet only about 10,000 years ago, and the human gut hasn't yet evolved to digest them properly. For 2.5 million years before grains were introduced, all the necessary nutrients the body needed were provided by eating animals from head to tail, vegetables, fruits, nuts, and seeds.

"Vegetable oils are healthy."

Consider This: Vegetable oils are mostly inflammatory and are chemically unstable. When they are introduced into the body, they potentially create serious health problems. In addition, chemically altered trans fats and partially hydrogenated fats are toxic to the body. Saturated fats from coconut oil, avocados, animals that are pastured and/or allowed to eat that natural diet, and butter from grass-fed cows are necessary for healthy cell function.

"Artificial sweeteners are good for you and help you lose weight."

Consider This: Artificial sweeteners are toxic to the body. In addition, the brain senses the sweetness of these sweeteners and stimulates insulin production.

"Eggs are bad for your heart."

Consider This: Free-range eggs provide excellent nutrition for the body unless you are allergic to eggs. Some people who have reactions to eggs from chickens that are confined to cages and fed an unnatural diet do not have a problem with eggs from pastured chickens. The cholesterol in pastured eggs is rarely a problem--especially if the egg yolk is eaten soft rather than scrambled or hard-boiled.

"If your stomach does not hurt, you don't have gut problems."

Consider This: Most disease begins when the intestinal lining becomes permeable (called a *leaky gut*), and stuff that should never enter the blood system starts invading. A person does not have to have digestive symptoms such as gas or pain or constipation or diarrhea to have a leaky gut. But, before other disease manifestations can be resolved, the gut must be made healthy.

And these are all *facts* you can take to the bank--the *food* bank!

24. Why the Tooth Fairies Gave Up Grains

I was once asked to write a story for an issue of *Care Magazine*® that would be appropriate for children and would answer some of their parents' questions about a healthy diet. My wife, who is the creative force in my life, came up with this whimsical idea for a title. Let your young kids read the story, which went something like this. Afterwards, discuss my questions and answers with them.

The story begins

You may think you know all about tooth fairies. You may know that they appear at night to exchange your baby teeth that your parents have tucked away under your pillow for little trinkets or even money. The tooth fairies flutter about the room as you sleep with their cute big eyes and their huge smiles and soft, silky wings. But what you probably *didn't* know was that these precious little busy bees have been around for a long time. As a matter of fact, they have been around for tens of thousands of years.

Something else you probably didn't know is that tooth fairies haven't always been so busy. In fact, there was a time when little boys and little girls hardly ever got tooth decay or lost their teeth from toothaches. In those days, mommies and daddies worked hard gathering and hunting for food. Their children ate all the good, nutritious foods that their parents brought to the table. Their young bodies were strong and lean, and their teeth were white and straight. Adult teeth lasted a lifetime, as they were designed to do. But then, something changed, even though the fairies didn't realize it until much later.

About 10 thousand years ago, farmers began to cultivate, or grow, certain plants to provide more food for people. Before long, these plants had become part of almost everyone's diet. The fairies didn't think any harm was going to come from these new foods. But it did. In time, these foods started to damage the teeth of little boys and girls--and their parents, too! All of a sudden, it seemed as if everyone began getting toothaches and cavities. They began losing their teeth. Finally, the fairies finally realized that something was wrong with these new foods. They discovered that these foods, called *grains*, were the cause of the dental problems and other health problems that were beginning to plague people around the world.

Then, refined sugar, corn syrup, and other sweeteners became part of most people's diets. The fairies at last began to understand that these sugars added to the problems from grains. The fairies made a pledge to give up these grains and sugars and to try to warn everybody else that these were *not* healthy foods.

So the fairies focused their goals on their new mission: to tell the world that grains and sugars needed to be avoided in order to regain healthy teeth and overall physical well-being. They understood that our bodies were never designed to eat these modern day foods. Our guts couldn't fully digest them, and the foods eventually upset our bodies' delicate balance. It took a long time for the fairies to realize that so many serious and long-lasting health problems were being caused by the new "processed foods."

So, the fairies gave up grains and sugars and started to make the world a better, healthier place in which to live. Most importantly, they set about teaching the young children of the world, whom they loved so much and wanted to protect from poor health, to eat healthier so they could enjoy life more.

Did they succeed? What do *you* think?

Parents' Q & A's

To create healthy meals for their children, parents need to leave grains and added-sugars out of their families' diets and to replace them with healthier food choices, including meats, fish, vegetables, fruit, nuts, seeds, and various spices. It's also important to eliminate unhealthy fats and to include leafy green vegetables at every meal. The foods that hunter-gatherers ate for thousands and thousands of years are the foods that will allow healthy bodies of all ages to survive and thrive today. These food choices are part of my *Lifestyle-Repair Plan.*

Q: Is a Primal diet a healthy diet for children under age 18?

A: Absolutely. But the term "diet" is misleading. A diet generally is a strict form of eating where calories are counted and portions of food are measured in some fashion. A Primal diet is really a lifestyle of eating nutrient-dense foods with no concern for calories. When the proper foods are eaten together, the body begins to regulate its digestive hormones, and the body will tell you to stop eating because it is full. Every meal should be thought of as a plate of food. Conceptually, at least one-half of the plate should consist of non-starchy vegetables; about one-quarter should consist of some type of protein; and the last quarter or less could be made up of additional healthy fats such as nuts or seeds or possibly a starchy vegetable or some deeply colored fruit. The nutrients that are available from eating animal products, vegetables, fruits, nuts, and seeds are all the nutrients that the human body needs--no matter what a person's age.

Q: Does some sugar in my child's diet mean they are destined for poor dental health?

A: Sugar in the natural form is not the same as concentrated sugars and refined sugars that are added to processed foods. Sugars that are in fruits are much healthier than the sugars a child gets in soda, sports drinks, cakes, cookies, candy, etc. However, if too much fresh fruit is eaten instead of balancing fruit with proteins, vegetables, and healthy fats, then too much fructose will affect the body, creating excesses for the liver and the brain, damaging the gut, and creating fat deposits around the waist. Sugar is a fermentable carbohydrate. If bad bacteria are predominant in the mouth and throughout the body, and if sugar is a dominant element in the child's diet, then tooth decay will be inevitable.

Q: How do you suggest dealing with the typical parent's dilemma of keeping sugary foods out of their children's diet? Regulating or eliminating sweets, sugary drinks, refined milk products, and processed grain treats sounds good in theory, but doing so isn't often practical in the real world. Often, I'm not even aware if my children are ingesting sugar... i.e. in a sports drink or an "energy" bar after a Little League game or even cakes, cookies, and ice cream at a birthday party.

A: Parents are in control of the foods that are presented to their children. Healthy foods are easy to provide, but in the beginning there is a learning curve. I have listed my favorite Paleo recipes later in the book.

The foods that are most important to eliminate are grains, added sugars, and unhealthy fats. Whole foods will not contribute significantly to an unhealthy sugar level. If a child's food choices in the home are generally healthy, then some cheating outside of the home is not going to be a problem.

The younger the child is when starting on a Primal lifestyle, the easier it will be to follow. An older child's eating habits may be more difficult to change but not impossible. Take baby steps, but remember: Children learn from what they see at home. *You* are their most important role model.

Q: We're so often in a hurry to get everything done in a typical day. Grocery shopping presents quite a hurdle. It's so much easier to "grab and go" when my kids are hungry and need to be fed. What's a parent to do?

A: Again, try to avoid the grains, added sugars, and unhealthy fats. Shop the outer aisles in the grocery store where the more natural foods are located and avoid the packaged and overly processed foods in the center of the store. If purchasing packaged foods, look at the ingredients, and be selective. You will be amazed at what are in some of these "foods." Again, grains, added sugars, and unhealthy fats are the most troublesome. You may not be 100% Primal, but you will be providing your child with a very healthy foundation. Some quick ideas for on-the-go feedings:

- Serve celery stalks with raw almond butter.
- Use raw fruit and vegetable slices for dipping in individual containers of live-culture, full-fat yogurt. Add spices or other natural flavors to the yogurt to create different taste sensations.
- Combine chicken salad or tuna salad (made with Healthy Mayo from my recipes in the back of the book) with chopped nuts, blueberries, and cut up celery. Lettuce leaves (butter or Romaine are healthy varieties) are good for a quick "sandwich wrap."
- Serve healthy raw macadamia nuts

Q: When we're traveling, are fast-food restaurants banned? What if we're on our way to an out-of-town game and can't take the time to stop for a sit down meal?

A: Fast food places usually are not a problem once you understand what you cannot eat. Some examples of your best food choices:

- Some type of salad with a homemade dressing of olive oil and vinegar and whatever spices are available at the restaurant.
- Hard boiled eggs, hamburger, or chicken meat, crumbled up and tossed into the salad for extra flavor and variety.
- Fresh fruit if available.
- Water, unsweetened iced or hot tea, or seltzer in place of soda or other sweetened drinks.

APPENDIX

i. The Preparation

Congratulations! You have been personally selected to take a tour of my private kitchen. I've tried to give you a good idea of what I use and how I use it while cooking.

Of course, this is only a guide for you. It's not set in stone. What works for me may not work for you. For example, you may have problems with cayenne pepper, which is not a problem for me. Obviously, you wouldn't stock cayenne pepper in your pantry.

You will most likely be spending more time in the kitchen preparing food than you have in the past, now that you know what you know. It will become fun. It has for me.

Certain items will become your staples based on your family's tastes. Prepare yourself for a kitchen experience. Don't be afraid to experiment; I often do. And remember, experiments do fail; they often have for me.

I like to have almost everything I need available in my kitchen. I can always go to the grocery store to buy an unusual item or items that I use up frequently, but the items below are the items that I try to keep on hand all the time.

Most of the items below are available at most grocery stores or online from Amazon. I am a shopper on Amazon because it is so easy, and most of the options are on the Amazon site in one place for me to make my decision. You also can set up regular shipments at the frequency you want for items you use up--for example: monthly, every 2 months, etc.

The gadgets that I suggest are the ones I use routinely; I would be lost without them. I have listed brand names for the ones that I think are exceptional or one-of-a-kind that gets the job done for me. It is always a matter of preference. As I said, what works for me may not work for you. However, this may be a perfect starting point for you.

Whenever I begin to start cooking, I always get everything that I will need for the recipe ready to go. That means all the ingredients are already out on the counter; veggies are already cleaned, cut, and prepared; proteins are unwrapped and defrosted if necessary; all gadgets are lined up. I am also prepared to cleanup as I go so that I don't have everything to clean up at the end. That's how I do it.

Just a reminder: Spices and food items are organic if possible. Animal products are also from pastured or wild caught sources, which have consumed only their natural diets with no chemicals or artificial ingredients added.

Spices

- Baking powder (aluminum free)
- Baking soda
- Basil
- Cacao powder
- Cayenne pepper
- Ceylon cinnamon
- Chili powder
- Chocolate extract
- Cloves
- Coarse salt
- Coffee extract
- Cumin
- Dry mustard
- Garlic powder
- Ginger
- Ground pepper
- Herbs de Provence
- Himalayan salt
- Oregano
- Paprika
- Parsley flakes
- Red pepper flakes
- Thyme
- Turmeric
- Vanilla pure extract

Refrigerator Foods

- Avocados
- Butter (Kerrygold® unsalted Irish Butter)
- Celery
- Cucumbers
- Dijon mustard
- Eggs
- Garlic
- Horseradish (Gold's prepared)
- Kimchi
- Leafy greens (kale, chard, spinach)
- Lemons
- Olives (black, green)
- Onions
- Sauerkraut (Bubbies)

Freezer Foods

- Bacon
- Bones for bone broth
- Chicken liver
- Chicken thighs (skin on and bone in)
- Ginger, fresh-cut into 1 inch pieces and then frozen
- Ground beef heart
- Ground beef, pork, lamb, veal
- Mussels
- Oxtail
- Shrimp
- Wild caught Pacific salmon

Pantry Foods

- Canned fish: anchovies
- Canned fish: clams
- Canned fish: salmon (canned, wild caught Pacific with skin and bones)

- Canned fish: sardines (canned, wild caught Pacific with skin and bones)
- Coconut aminos
- Diced and fire roasted tomatoes with green chilies in can
- Local raw honey
- Maple syrup or Molasses
- Nut flour: almond flour
- Nut flour: coconut flour
- Nuts: almonds, raw
- Nuts: macadamia nuts, raw
- Oil: avocado oil
- Oil: coconut oil
- Oil: extra virgin olive oil for salads
- Oil: light olive oil for mayo
- Oil: macadamia oil
- Oil: red palm oil
- Seaweed: dulse flakes (Maine Coast)
- Seaweed: kelp granules
- Seaweed: Pacific kombu (Emerald Cove)
- Seaweed: Pacific wakame (Emerald Cove)
- Teas (green, black, white, hibiscus, matcha)
- Tomato paste
- Unmodified potato starch (resistant starch)
- Vinegar: Apple cider vinegar (unfiltered)
- Vinegar: Balsamic vinegar
- Vinegar: Rice vinegar
- Worcestershire sauce

Gadgets

- Apron (Chef Works AB041-BLK-0 Bronx Bib Apron, Black)
- Avocado slicer
- Baking sheet
- BlenderVitamix (powerful and has 8-cup capacity but no storage container)

- NutriBullet Rx (has smaller capacity than Vitamix but more convenient, easier to clean, and the containers double as storage containers--a big convenience)
- Can opener
- Cheesecloth (great for filtering ghee)
- Chopping knife
- Citrus juicer (manual)
- Coffee grinder
- Coffee maker (French press)
- Colander
- Flexible cutting mats
- Flexible measuring cups and funnel
- Food chopper: hand
- Food processor
- Glass containers with airtight lids which can store in freezer, can be heated in oven without lid, and can be used to serve from
- Jar Opener: Gripper (Kuhn Rikon®)
- Kitchen scissors
- Knife, Chef (OXO Good Grips Professional 6-1/2-Inch Santoku Knife)
- Knife, serrated utility 5-inch
- Lemon/lime manual squeezer
- Mandolin
- Mason jars
- Measuring cups (Pyrex: 1-cup, 4-cup)
- Measuring spoons
- Organic coffee filter to make ghee or cheesecloth bag or cheesecloth to line funnel
- Pots and Pans (I like the CTX ScanPan® family which is a ceramic titanium surface on stainless steel)
  - 3.7 qt covered sauce pan
  - 10 1/4" covered sauté pan
  - 12 1/2" covered sauté pan
  - 5.1 qt covered Dutch oven

- Salad spinner
- Silicone muffin mold
- Slow cooker
- Spatulas (silicone and wood)
- Splatter screen
- Stainless steel box grater
- Steamer pot (3-quart, covered, stainless steel)
- Stick blender or handheld mixer
- Storage containers and travel containers for smoothies (BPA free or stainless steel)
- Strainer for bone broth (Winco CCB-8 Bouillon Strainer, 8-Inch Diameter, Extra Fine Mesh)
- Tongs (silicone)

Disposables

- Aluminum foil (to line the bottom of the oven to catch drippings)
- Parchment paper
- Plastic wrap
- Storage bag (Ziplock: 1-quart and 1-gallon sizes)
- Toothpicks to check doneness of muffins and custards

ii. What I Eat

Here is a sample of a typical day's food for me. I don't eat these items every day. I eat when I am hungry; I stop when I am satisfied; I drink when I am thirsty. Sometimes I eat breakfast; frequently I don't. I practice intermittent fasting as I have described in previous chapters. These work for me. Again, eat when you are hungry; stop when you are satisfied. Our primal ancestors did not eat breakfast, lunch, and dinner with in-between snacks on a scheduled basis. Our guts need a rest for proper digestion.

Breakfast

Eggs over easy with organic greens (kale, chard, spinach, or arugula) sautéed in ghee or grass-fed butter or coconut oil seasoned with sea salt, pepper, and kelp granules.

OR

Smoothie with 1/2 cup fresh-frozen blueberries, 1/2 frozen banana (I freeze my very ripe bananas), 2 cups raw organic greens (dandelion, kale, chard, spinach, or beet greens), 1 avocado, 2-3 cups water, and sometimes 1 or 2 raw egg yolks from pastured chickens and sometimes 1/2 tsp. cinnamon. Blend until smooth in heavy-duty blender such as a Vitamix blender[239] or NutriBullet Rx[240]. *YUM!*

OR

Most often I will skip breakfast if I am not hungry (i.e.: intermittent fasting) and eat my first meal between noon and 2 p.m. In the morning I often will drink my spiced rendition of Dave Asprey's BulletProof® Coffee, which is in my Recipes at the end of the book.

Lunch

Could be what I suggested for breakfast above.

OR

Raw organic bell pepper (green, red, orange, or yellow sliced in half with seeds removed) stuffed with canned wild salmon or sardines (including bones and skin) with lime juice and ground pistachios sprinkled on top.

Dinner

Sautéed organic greens (kale, chard, spinach, or dandelion), fresh garlic, and organic onions in coconut oil or Ghee; seasoned with turmeric, sea salt, and pepper; finished off with a few organic raisins, freshly squeezed lime or lemon juice, and slivered almonds.

Grass-fed burgers (veal, beef, or buffalo) mixed with organic Jalapeno peppers, organic onions, sea salt, pepper, and garlic powder

OR

Wild-caught salmon baked in parchment paper with ghee and seasoned with sea salt, pepper, lemon juice, and Herbs de Provence.

Snacks

Raw macadamia nuts, berries and citrus in season

Dark chocolate (I really like 85% Dark Blackout Organic Chocolate by Alter Eco: www.alterecofoods.com).

And every day:

I like to include sauerkraut or kimchi with at least one meal because of the taste and the probiotics. I try to include my smoothie with many meals. I drink plain water as well as kombucha and green or herbal teas, such as Japanese Ceremonial Matcha Green Tea for a very special and healthy drink (www.MatchaSource.com or www.Teavana.com). I also like to consume bone broth made from pastured animal bones, which has significant health benefits. Before bed I may take a soil-based probiotic that I already described (Prescript Assist®) and some resistant starch (unmodified potato starch) dissolved in a glass of water.

Now you're *cookin'!*

I have experimented with lots of recipes over the years. I love to cook now, but I never cooked before I became immersed in a primal lifestyle and a primal way of eating. The recipes that are in this chapter are the ones that I make most frequently for my wife and me. I prepare all these delights at least a few times a month. They are easy, but you will have a learning curve to make them the way that is best for you and your family. The way I describe them is the way I make them in my kitchen. We love them just as they are written in the following pages. You may want to tweak the ingredients or their proportions based on your tastes.

I often prepare most of the main dishes on the weekend in sufficient quantities so that I have plenty to freeze for later use. Then during the week, I prepare smoothies that I drink daily and vegetable dishes to serve with the previously frozen main courses.

I have divided this section into five main categories: Drinks, Desserts, Sides and Main, Dishes, Special Dishes, and Miscellaneous. All ingredients are either organic or grown locally or purchased from my local CSA (Community Supported Agriculture) store. Similarly, all animal products come from pastured and naturally fed animals. No grain-fed animal products and no commercially raised animals (CAFO, or Concentrated Animal Feeding Operation) are allowed. Also, all fish and shellfish are from wild-caught sources.

A couple other points worth noting as you prepare your kitchen for your new health lifestyle:

- When using coconut oil, you need to be aware that it is a solid below 76°F. It should be liquefied before using to make it easier to incorporate into recipes. It is best to slightly heat it in a saucepan on the stove, or you could use a warm stainless steel spoon to scoop it out of the container and put it in a warmed Pyrex measuring cup to allow the coconut oil to further soften and melt.

- When sautéing with any oils or ghee, be aware they will most likely splatter. I always use a splatter screen, and I always wear an apron. (I've ruined too many good shirts and pants. Now I know better!)
- All nuts and seeds should be soaked overnight in warm, salty water using sea salt. In the morning, rinse the nuts and seeds. You could allow them to dry to use later, or you could use them wet right away.
- Be aware that some of my recipes include nut flours, honey, and fruits that are high in carbohydrates. They should be used sparingly! Recipes on the Internet that are touted as "Paleo" and include nut flours, starches, and dried fruits are not okay to eat regularly on a Paleo diet. These recipes are high in carbohydrates and are not healthy. They could significantly increase weight and boost other markers of metabolic syndrome.

One final word

So...at last. Here we are. My big question to you now is, are you ready to get started? The recipes in the next section will help launch you into an exciting new world of culinary delight and sweep you off into a brand new direction toward a stronger, healthier lifestyle. *Bon appétit!*

iii. The Recipes
Drinks

Gazpacho with Watermelon and Spicy Tomato

This is a refreshing version of gazpacho with a sweet and spicy kick. I first read of it by Michelle Tam from Nom Nom Paleo[241], and then I tweaked the ingredients for my taste.

Ingredients:

- 2 cans (14.5 oz. each) diced and fire roasted organic tomatoes with green chilies
- 1 cucumber
- 2 small shallots, coarsely chopped
- 1 celery stalk
- 1 pound seedless watermelon (approximately 3 cups)
- 2 tablespoons apple cider vinegar
- 1/3 cup extra virgin olive oil
- Salt and pepper to taste
- Pinch of red pepper flakes (optional)

Preparation:

- Peel the cucumber and cut into pieces
- Place tomatoes, cucumber, shallots, and celery into a large power blender (in use a Vitamix for this recipe)
- Blend until puréed.
- Once the veggies are liquefied, add the watermelon, vinegar, olive oil and blend until smooth.
- Salt and pepper to taste and if necessary blend some more
- Add a pinch of red pepper flakes if you want some more heat, and blend some more
- Refrigerate the soup until it's fully chilled
- Ladle the gazpacho into cups or bowls, and enjoy

Hot Cocoa

Do you remember drinking hot chocolate on a cold day to make the chill go away? What a great excuse to have a hot chocolate. Most hot chocolate drinks were loaded with table sugar, milk, and some type of processed chocolate mix that included ingredients that were artificial and not so healthy. Here is a recipe that is the real deal. Try it; you might like it--hot cocoa as it was meant to be. And, very healthy, too.

Cocoa is the spicy powder that makes chocolate taste like chocolate. It is one of the richest sources of flavanols. Studies have shown that flavanols can disarm cell-damaging free radicals, preserve cell membranes, protect DNA, prevent the formation of artery-clogging plaque, improve blood flow to the heart, lower high blood pressure, and prevent blood clots that can cause a heart attack or stroke.

Most chocolate drinks contain milk. Be aware that milk can bind to the flavanols in cocoa interfering with their absorption by the body.

There are two surprises in this recipe: ghee and Pastured Egg Yolk. Both will give the drink body and smoothness. Ghee is made from the butter of grass-fed cows and is all butterfat with no milk solids (my recipe for ghee is in this section). The pastured egg yolk will add significant nutrients to the drink. If you included some sautéed greens as a side dish with this drink, you would have a great meal.

Ingredients:
- 1 1/2 tablespoons unsweetened organic cocoa powder
- 1 tablespoon raw, local honey
- 1 tablespoon ghee
- 1/2 teaspoon vanilla extract
- 1/4 teaspoon ground cinnamon
- Pinch of ground cloves
- 1 pastured egg yolk
- 8 ounces hot water (not boiling)

Preparation:

- Mix all ingredients together and blend with a stick blender
- Yum!

Spiced BulletProof Coffee

Dave Asprey introduced his BulletProof Coffee several years ago, and it has become extremely popular. Here is a link to his website and recipe for his BulletProof Coffee[242]. Below is my spiced version that I love and drink almost every morning. There are interesting health benefits from coffee, coconut oil, ghee from the butter of grass-fed cows, cinnamon, and organic cocoa. It is easy to make your own ghee, and my ghee recipe is in this chapter.

If your body is not used to these quantities of healthy fats, you must start slowly. Use only 1-2 teaspoons of the coconut oil as well as the ghee at first. Also, start with only 1 teaspoon of cinnamon and cocoa. Gradually increase the amounts until you reach what works for you. These measures are what I use for myself.

You will need a basic blender to get the mixture to froth. I use a stick blender (Cuisinart Hand Blender), which has worked well for me.

Ingredients:

- 5-6 Tbs freshly ground organic coffee beans (I like shade-grown, organic Ethiopian beans)
- 16 oz filtered water
- 2 Tbs organic virgin coconut oil - start with 1 teaspoon
- 2 Tbs ghee made from butter of grass-fed cows - start with 1 teaspoon
- 1 Tbs organic cocoa powder - start with 1 teaspoon
- 1 Tbs ground Ceylon cinnamon - start with 1 teaspoon (Ceylon cinnamon is different than Cassia types of cinnamon[243]. Cassia types are the ones mostly sold in grocery stores.)

Preparation:

- Grind beans to coarse-grind and use French Press
- Place ground beans in French Press and add water that has come to a boil and cooled for 1 minute; then brew for 4 minutes
- While coffee is brewing, add coconut oil, ghee, cocoa powder, and cinnamon into 32 ounce Pyrex cup so you have plenty of room to mix with the blender
- Press brewed coffee after 4 minutes of steeping and pour hot coffee into measuring cup
- Blend mixture until well mixed and frothy
- Put into Thermos-type container to keep warm, and enjoy!

Spiced BulletProof Matcha

Matcha is stoneground green tea leaves and a Japanese delicacy. It provides a powerful arsenal of vitamins, minerals, antioxidants, fiber, chlorophyll and amino acids in a way no other green tea can. One glass of matcha is equivalent to 10 glasses of green tea in terms of nutritional value and antioxidant content. It has a unique spinach-like taste.

Here is a recipe I created. It is like my Spiced BulletProof Coffee that is based on Dave Asprey's BulletProof Coffee. If you need sweetness, you could add some raw honey. I have included an optional topping of whipped coconut cream. Play with the quantities, and settle with what tastes best for you. Start off with the least amount of ghee and coconut oil so that your system gets used to these fats. Also, experiment with the cocoa and cinnamon amounts.

You can find more information about matcha at on this website.[244] You also could order various qualities of matcha from this company.

Ingredients:

- 2 teaspoons matcha powder
- 12 oz filtered water (just off boil)
- 1-2 Tsp organic virgin coconut oil
- 1-2 Tsp ghee or unsalted butter (made from grass-fed cows)
- 1 Tsp organic cocoa powder
- 1 Tsp ground Ceylon cinnamon
- Raw honey (optional)

Optional topping:

- 1 can coconut milk (use cream that separated from coconut milk and discard liquid)
- 1 tsp vanilla extract

Preparation:

- Place matcha powder in 4-cup Pyrex measuring cup
- Add hot water, coconut oil, ghee, cocoa powder, and cinnamon and blend with power mixer (stick blender)
- Blend mixture until well mixed and frothy
- Optional: add raw honey

Preparation of optional topping:

- Place can of coconut milk upside down into freezer for 5 minutes, which allows the cream to solidify on top and separate from the liquid on the bottom. Open other end, pour off liquid, and remove cream.
- Place coconut cream into separate mixing bowl; add vanilla and whip until consistency of whipped cream
- Place whipped coconut cream on top of hot matcha blend

Yummy and Oh-So-Healthy Smoothie

Leafy greens are so important for the micronutrients your body's cells require to function efficiently and effectively. Sometimes it may seem difficult to eat prepared or raw greens with every meal, as you should. However, if the greens are reduced into a drink, it might be easier to include them with meals.

I drink smoothies every day. I may substitute different berries for the blueberries. I will vary some of the leafy greens. I may use a couple of raw egg yolks instead of the avocado. In addition to the following recipe, I sometimes include beets, carrots, celery, or other veggies for variety. But, I always have the majority of the smoothie consisting of leafy greens. Below is my basic, healthy drink. Try it out. You just may fall in love with it as I have.

Ingredients:

- Swiss chard
- Kale
- Spinach
- Blueberries
- Avocado (peeled and pitted)
- Banana (peeled)

Preparation:

- Use a good blender, which is essential (examples: Vitamix, NutriBullet Rx)
- Pack a mixture of Swiss chard, kale, and spinach into the blender to the half-full mark
- Add the banana and blueberries up to the 2/3 full mark
- Add avocado
- Add enough cold water to cover the contents
- Blend at high speed until all contents are fully liquefied
- If more "sweetness" is required, add more blueberries and/or banana
- Store in refrigerator and drink with meals

Desserts

Baked Custard

Creamy and delicious--great dessert. If you cannot find coconut cream, you can place 3, 15.5-oz cans of coconut milk in the freezer for 5 minutes upside down. The cream will solidify and separate from the remaining liquid. Turn the can right side up, and open. Discard the liquid and use the cream.

Ingredients:

- 2-cups full-fat coconut cream (Native Forest is organic and does not have BPA in the lining of their cans) or 2-cups raw heavy whipping cream
- 5 egg yolks
- 1/4 cup local, raw honey
- 2 teaspoons vanilla extract
- Optional: Nutmeg, cinnamon, or other spice of your choosing

Preparation:

- Preheat oven to 350°F
- Warm the cream up on the stove over low heat.
- While the cream is heating on the stove, mix the 5 egg yolks with the honey and vanilla in a separate bowl with a hand mixer until smooth.
- Prepare 6 custard dishes by placing them in a baking dish large enough to hold them along with a water bath.
- When the cream is hot to the touch of your finger (but not boiling), slowly pour it into the egg/honey mixture while mixing; blend well.
- Pour into custard dishes, and fill the baking dish with hot water up to 1/2 to 2/3 of the height of the custard dishes so it acts as a bath.
- Sprinkle with ground nutmeg and/or cinnamon
- Bake at 350°F for about 50 minutes until a toothpick inserted in the center comes out clean.
- Remove from water bath immediately and let cool.

Banana Bread Supreme

I have tried many banana bread recipes, but this one is the best.[245] Most Paleo-type recipes usually have been very dry to my taste. This has been moist and reminiscent of the banana breads I have enjoyed before going Primal. Go easy. This is a treat; not a regular part of my diet.

Ingredients

- 4 bananas, yellow
- 4 eggs
- 1/2 cup almond butter (or any nut butter, i.e. macadamia, pecan, etc.)
- 4 tablespoons ghee or liquefied coconut oil
- 1/2 cup coconut flour
- 1 Tbs cinnamon
- 1 Tsp baking soda
- 1 Tsp baking powder
- 1 Tsp vanilla
- 1/8 Tsp sea salt

Preparation:

- Preheat your oven to 350°F
- Combine bananas, eggs, and nut butter, and ghee or coconut oil in a Vitamix, Nutribullet Rx, or food processor and mix well
- Add coconut flour, cinnamon, baking soda, baking powder, vanilla, and sea salt and mix well
- Grease a 9×5 glass loaf pan with coconut oil
- Pour in batter, and place in oven
- Bake for 55-60 minutes (until a toothpick inserted into the center comes out clean)
- Remove from oven and flip out onto a cooling rack
- Slice and serve

Blueberry Muffins

If I would have a muffin, it would be a blueberry muffin with a bunch of plump blueberries oozing out from all directions. This is a great Paleo recipe with lots of blueberries, but it is heavy on carbs - about 35 grams of carbs per muffin. They are to be eaten as a treat. This recipe makes 6 muffins.

Ingredients:

Dry:

- 1 cup almond flour
- 6 Tbs Arrowroot powder
- 1/4 tsp salt

Wet:

- 1 egg
- 1/4 cup raw honey
- 1/4 cup coconut oil
- 2 tsp vanilla extract
- 1 cup blueberries (fresh organic or frozen and thawed with excess liquid drained off)

Preparation:

- Preheat oven to 350° F
- Combine dry ingredients in a large mixing bowl
- In a separate mixing bowl, combine wet ingredients
- Add wet ingredients to dry ingredients and stir
- Add vanilla extract
- Add blueberries
- Place in muffin cups and bake for 20-25 minutes. I actually use a silicone mold that I purchased at Disneyworld. Can you guess the shape of my muffins?

Chewy, Chocolaty Brownies

My weakness forever has been chewy, yummy, rich, chocolate brownies. In the past, these were very unhealthy and definitely not Paleo. Then I found a recipe that I tweaked to make it my favorite brownie recipe--even better than the non-Paleo types. So, if you love brownies as I did and still do, then you must try this recipe. Remember, this is an indulgence--not meant to be eaten every day. (One-square equals about 22 grams of carbs.)

Ingredients:

- 1 cup raw honey
- 3/4 cup organic cocoa powder
- 1 cup almond butter
- 1 pastured egg
- 2 tsp vanilla extract
- 1 tsp chocolate extract
- 1 tsp coffee extract
- 1/2 tsp baking powder
- 1/2 tsp salt

Preparation:

- Heat honey gently over stove until warm; do not boil. (If you want a sweeter brownie, you could add an additional 1/4-cup of honey. If you want less sweetness, reduce the recipe to 3/4 cup raw honey.)
- Stir in cocoa powder over low heat until smooth. Cocoa burns easily, so keep the heat on very low.
- Remove from heat and stir in almond butter.
- In separate bowl: mix egg, vanilla, chocolate and coffee extracts, and baking powder.
- Add to honey/cocoa/almond butter mixture and stir batter until smooth
- Sprinkle batter with salt, and fold batter to incorporate salt.
- Pour into parchment-paper-lined 8x8 baking pan, or grease the pan with coconut oil.
- Bake brownies at 325° F for 35-45 minutes.
- Insert a toothpick in the center of brownies to determine if done.
- Let cool completely before cutting.
- Cut into 2-inch squares (total 16 pieces).
- Store extras in freezer and thaw when ready for another.

Chocolate Coconut Nut Balls

Great ingredients for a great dessert. Macadamia nuts are probably the healthiest of all nuts.

Ingredients:

- 1 Cup macadamia nuts
- 1 Tbs coconut flour
- 3 Tbs local, raw honey
- 2 Tbs coconut oil
- 3 Tbs cocoa powder
- 1 Tbs zest of orange
- 1/8 Tsp sea salt
- 1 C shredded unsweetened coconut

Preparation:

- Place nuts, flour, honey, coconut oil, cocoa powder, orange zest, and salt in a food processor and pulse until formed into a thick mixture
- Roll into 1-inch balls
- Roll each ball in shredded coconut to cover
- Refrigerate

Pumpkin Muffins

Although these muffins[246] are moist and delicious, they do have fructose in the form of honey for sweetness (total carbs about 11 grams per muffin). So, discretion is important. You could leave out the honey or reduce the quantity in order to reduce the amount of carbohydrates, but you will sacrifice sweetness. You need to experiment, but honey is a whole food. This recipe should make 12 muffins.

Ingredients:

- 1 1/2 cups almond flour
- 3/4 cup canned organic pumpkin
- 3 large free-range eggs
- 1/8 tsp sea salt
- 1 tsp baking soda
- 1 tsp baking powder
- 1/2 tsp cinnamon

- 1 1/2 tsp pumpkin pie spice
- 1/4 cup raw, local honey
- 2 tsp almond butter

Preparation:

- Preheat oven to 350° F
- Coat muffin mold with coconut oil
- Mix all ingredients until smooth, and pour evenly into mold
- Bake for 25 minutes on the middle rack (check with a toothpick to see if done)

Zucchini Brownies[247] with Dark Chocolate Icing

No veggie taste here--just great chocolate! These brownies are moist and chocolaty with a luscious dark chocolate icing if you are so inclined. Remember, these are treats and not for every day.

Ingredients for Brownies:

- 2 cups zucchini, thinly chopped
- 1 cup almond butter
- 2 2.82 oz (80 gram) 85% dark chocolate bars (broken into small pieces)--my favorite dark chocolate bar is Dark Blackout Organic Chocolate by Alter Eco
- 1 egg
- 1/3 cup raw honey
- 1/4 cup organic applesauce
- 2 tsp. vanilla extract
- 1 tsp chocolate extract
- 1 tsp coffee extract
- 3 tbsp. cocoa powder
- 1 tsp. baking powder

Ingredients for Icing (optional):

- 1 1/2 2.82 oz (80 gram) 85% dark chocolate bars (broken into small pieces)
- 1/3 cup coconut oil
- 1 tablespoon vanilla extract

Preparation of Brownies:

- Preheat oven to 350° F.
- In a Vitamix or food processor or other power blender, combine all the ingredients for the brownies and mix.
- Pour the brownie mixture into a pan greased with coconut oil.
- Place in the oven and bake for 40-45 minutes.
- Check for doneness with a toothpick in the center of the brownies.
- Wait until the brownies are cool before cutting and removing from the pan. (If placing icing, cut after placing icing)

Preparation of Icing (optional):

- Combine the broken dark chocolate bars and coconut oil in a pan on the stove.
- Heat over low heat until melted and stir in the vanilla.
- Allow to cool completely
- Whip with a hand mixer until fluffy.
- Spread over cooled brownies before cutting. (Top with fresh berries for a special treat)

Sides/Main Dishes

Blueberry Chutney

Chutney can be almost anything. Basically, it's a spicy condiment originating in India and made of fruits or vegetables with vinegar, spices, and something sweet. Here is delicious chutney that can be a tasty topping for many different foods or eaten by itself.

Ingredients:

- 2 cups organic blueberries
- 1 cup chopped onion
- 2 Tbsp. balsamic vinegar
- 2 Tbsp. raisins

- 1/2 Tbsp. ginger powder
- 1/2 Tbsp. garlic powder
- 1/2 Tbsp. cinnamon
- 1/4 tsp. sea salt
- 1-2 Tbsp. fresh chopped mint (optional)

Preparation:

- Combine all of the ingredients in a small saucepan and bring to a boil.
- Reduce the heat and simmer, stirring occasionally, until thickened (30-40 min).
- Allow to cool, and then add the mint if desired.
- Serve over a variety of meats and seafood, or eat it by itself.

Broccoli Coconut Puree

Soup and winter months go so well together. Actually, anytime is great for soup. This puree could be served hot or cold. When it comes to nourishment, broccoli is one of those nutrient-dense foods. It contains high levels of fiber (both soluble and insoluble) and is a rich source of vitamin-C. About 1-cup of raw broccoli florets provides around 110% of the recommended daily intake of vitamin C. Broccoli is also rich in vitamin A, iron, vitamin K, B-complex vitamins, zinc, phosphorus, phytonutrients and antioxidants. In addition, it has a good amount of protein for a non-starchy vegetable. Along with the other goodies in this recipe, how could you go wrong?

Think about garnishing with a couple of shrimp and/or some chopped, crispy bacon pieces. It's even thick enough to use cold as a dip for cucumbers or carrot sticks or whatever suits you.

Ingredients:

- 1 small sweet onion
- 1 small sweet potato
- 2 bunches of steamed broccoli florets (approximately 4 cups raw florets)
- 1 can coconut milk (13.5 oz.)

- 1/2 tsp Himalayan salt
- Pepper to taste

Preparation:

- Steam broccoli and onion for about 5 minutes
- Cook the sweet potato with the skin by steaming or in the oven at 350°F until tender
- After broccoli, onion, and sweet potato have cooled, cut them into small pieces and place in a powerful blender such as the Vitamix or the Nutribullet Rx
- Add coconut milk and salt and blend until hot and smooth
- Add pepper to taste and enjoy

Brussels Sprouts and Shrimp

Brussels sprouts are leafy green cruciferous vegetables that contain high levels of vitamins C and K, with moderate amounts of folate and vitamin B6 along with minerals and dietary fiber. Brussels sprouts also contain sulforaphane, a phytochemical that is reported to have anticancer properties, and indole-3-carbinol, a chemical that may help DNA repair in cells and may block the growth of cancer cells in. Boiling will reduce the level of sulforaphane, but steaming and stir frying will not result in a significant loss.

This recipe will take some preparation, but the results are delicious. You will need two saucepans.

Ingredients:

Onions and sauce in first saucepan

- 1/4 cup ghee
- 1 cup onion, chopped
- 1 tsp red pepper flakes
- 4 cloves garlic, minced
- 1/4 cup chopped parsley
- Juice of 1/2 lemon
- 1/4 cup red wine

- 1-2 Tsp raw honey

Brussels sprouts and shrimp in the second saucepan

- 1/4 cup ghee or coconut oil
- 2 cups Brussels sprouts sliced in half
- Salt and pepper to taste
- 1 pound shrimp, thawed and peeled

Preparation:

In the first pan

- Heat 1/4 cup ghee over medium-low heat
- Add onions, red pepper flakes, garlic and cook covered over medium-low heat until onions are soft.
- Add parsley and mix.
- Add wine and lemon juice and continue to heat uncovered to thicken.
- Drizzle honey and blend.
- Cover and set aside to use over shrimp and Brussels sprouts.

In the second pan

- Add 1/4 cup ghee or coconut oil over medium heat.
- Add Brussels sprouts to cook uncovered until slightly brown. (You may need to place a mesh splatter screen over pan to prevent splattering.)
- Salt and pepper to taste.
- Add shrimp and cook uncovered until translucent--only about 1-2 minutes. (Be careful not to overcook or the shrimp will be tough and rubbery).
- Pour reduced onion and garlic sauce over shrimp and Brussels sprouts.
- Plate and Enjoy!

Cauliflower Mash

Mashed potatoes used to be a great side dish for me. But, it was not Paleo since potatoes are high in carbs, relatively low in nutrients, and contain high levels of glycoalkaloids. Then I discovered mashed cauliflower, which could be made with the consistency and satisfaction of mashed potatoes without the bad stuff. Cauliflower is a cruciferous vegetable that has numerous health benefits. The kelp granules add necessary trace nutrients that are missing in most dishes.

Ingredients:

- 2 10-oz bags of cauliflower florets
- 2-3 Tbs ghee or butter from grass-fed cows
- Salt, pepper, garlic powder to taste
- 1 tsp organic kelp granules

Preparation:

- Cut florets into small pieces
- Place cauliflower into steamer pot to steam
- Turn burner on and steam cauliflower for 12-14 minutes (do not overcook)
- Place steamed cauliflower into Vitamix or food processor and blend until smooth
- Add fat, salt, pepper, garlic powder, and kelp granules-- adjust amounts for personal taste
- Eat as is or enjoy with toppings

Cauliflower Rice

This is a great substitute for white rice. White rice has lectins that may be a problem for some people. In addition, white rice has a high carbohydrate density (28.3%). A healthier vegetable would be cauliflower. Cauliflower has significantly more nutrition than white rice and has a lower carbohydrate density (1.8%). Try this in place of steamed rice.

Ingredients:

- 1 bag of cauliflower florets
- 1 tablespoon coconut oil
- 1 medium sweet onion, diced
- Himalayan salt and ground black pepper to taste

Preparation:

- Make sure cauliflower florets are dry
- Heat coconut oil in sauté pan to medium heat.
- Add onion and sauté approximately 10 minutes or until soft.
- Place cauliflower into food processor and "pulse" until cauliflower is small and has the texture of regular white rice. Don't over process. If you over process the cauliflower, it will get mushy.
- Raise the heat in the sauté pan to medium-high, and add the cauliflower "rice".
- Cover and cook approximately 5 to 6 minutes, stirring frequently, until the cauliflower is slightly crispy on the outside but tender on the inside.
- Season with salt and pepper to taste.
- Remove from heat and serve.

Variation Ideas:

You can get very creative. You might consider adding turmeric or other spices and herbs as the "rice" is cooking. You even could create "Chinese fried rice" by adding a beaten egg to the sauté pan after removing the "rice"; scramble the egg in the remaining oil in the sauté pan and add some coconut aminos. Then add back the rice and mix well.

Chicken Liver & Onions

Liver and onions were some of the foods my Mom served when I was a kid. Only it was beef liver that was always overdone and rubbery. I did not develop a taste for liver and onions. When I first tried chicken liver, it took some getting used to. Then, over the years I became a big fan of liver pâté. The secret to cooking liver is to never overcook it. Liver should be made medium rare so that it is soft and tasty.

Here's a very tasty recipe. After you eat the liver and onions, and if you have any leftovers, it is great to put it in a food processor and make pâté. Then, refrigerate it and have it for several more meals.

You might want to put 1-2 hardboiled eggs in the food processor after the liver and onions are pureed and chop the eggs to incorporate them into the liver pâté, resembling the traditional Jewish dish of chopped liver.

Ingredients:

- 1 Tbs ghee or coconut oil
- 1 small sweet onion, sliced thin
- 3 cloves garlic, chopped
- Salt and pepper to taste
- 1 lb chicken liver (washed and cut into halves)
- 2 tsp basil
- 1/4 cup red wine

Preparation:

- Add ghee or coconut oil to pan and heat to medium
- Add onions and sauté over medium heat (a splatter screen will help to prevent oil splatter)
- Add garlic and salt/pepper to taste; then cook on low heat to soften garlic
- Add livers to pan, again add salt and pepper to taste, and brown on both sides (medium rare)
- Add basil and wine and cook for another minute
- Adjust salt and pepper if necessary
- Serve warm

Chili with 4 Meats

I often make this dish on the weekend and freeze portions to use during the week. I created this, and I must confess that it is delicious. It combines some of the best tastes of several meats with healthy ground beef heart--this is a great way to include organ meats for those who are not used to them. The black garlic is fermented garlic that adds a unique sweet taste. I purchase this from my local Trader Joes when they have it in stock. You could easily purchase black garlic online if you can't find it in your healthy food store.

Ingredients:
- 1 lb bacon cut into 1/2 inch pieces
- 1 lb ground pork
- 1 lb ground beef
- 1 lb ground beef heart
- 1 package black garlic (1.75 oz) - mashed
- 1 large onion - chopped
- 1 lb cremini mushrooms - quartered
- 1 can of organic fire roasted tomatoes with organic green chilies (14.5 oz can)
- 1 can organic tomato paste (6 oz can)
- Salt and pepper to taste

Preparation:
- Begin to cook bacon in medium-heated large covered saucepan until liquefied fat is forming
- Add ground beef, pork, and heart to saucepan and brown; stir frequently
- Remove meat with slotted spoon (to allow fat to remain in pan), and place meat in large bowl
- Use meat fats in saucepan to sauté onions until translucent
- Add mashed black garlic to onions and mix thoroughly
- Add mushrooms and sauté until mushrooms have released their moisture and allow liquid to boil off
- Add meat mixture into pan with onions and mushrooms and blend well
- Add fire roasted tomatoes and tomato paste to saucepan and blend
- Simmer 10 - 15 minutes covered, and salt and pepper to taste

- Eat what you want now; you can freeze remaining portions in separate glass containers to reheat and serve during the week

Crab Imperial in Portobello Mushroom Caps

One of my favorite seafood dishes has been crab imperial. In Baltimore where I grew up, great crab dishes were common. Unfortunately, most crab imperial recipes use breading and other non-Paleo ingredients in the mixture. Here is my arrangement to fit my Paleo lifestyle.

There are 3 steps to this recipe:

1. Ingredients for Large Portobello Mushroom Caps:

- 4 large Portobello mushrooms
- 4 Tbs butter or ghee
- Salt and Pepper to taste
- Parchment paper and baking sheet

Preparation:

- Preheat oven to 350° F.
- Remove the stem (you also may want to scoop out some of the gills to make more room for crab mixture).
- Melt the butter or ghee in a large saucepan on medium and place the mushroom caps.
- Sauté for about 5 minutes on each side. You'll see that they'll flatten out and start to look brownish. Add salt and pepper to taste.
- Place on parchment paper that lines a baking sheet (cookie sheet).

2. Ingredients for Crab Mixture:

- 3 free-range eggs
- 1 Tbs parsley
- 1 tsp mustard (wet)
- 1/3 cup mayonnaise (my Healthier Mayo)
- Few drops Worcestershire sauce

235

- 1 lb lump crabmeat (drain excess water)

Preparation:

- Combine the eggs, parsley, mustard, mayonnaise, and Worcestershire in a small mixing bowl and blend well.
- Place the crabmeat in the mixing bowl. Gently combine the ingredients.
- Spoon the crabmeat mixture on top of the mushroom caps gill-side up (already on the parchment paper lined trays).
- There will be extra crab mixture which can be placed in a baking glass container to bake along with the stuffed mushroom caps
- Bake at 350° F for 15 minutes.

3. Ingredients for Topping:

- 6 tbs. mayonnaise (my Healthier Mayo), or plain full-fat yogurt (I like **7 Stars Farm** brand of yogurt)
- 1/2 tsp. Old Bay Seafood Seasoning
- 1/2 tsp. fresh lemon juice
- 1/2 tsp. Worcestershire Sauce
- Sprinkling of paprika

Preparation:

- While the crab is cooking, combine topping ingredients (mayonnaise or yogurt, seafood seasoning, lemon juice & Worcestershire sauce) in a medium mixing bowl and whip until smooth.
- After crab is finished baking, remove from oven and switch oven to broil.
- Top each baked crab imperial with the topping and a sprinkling of paprika.
- Place in broiler to finish off until imperials start to brown.
- Serve hot

Crispy Italian-spice Chicken Thighs

I used to love Southern fried chicken, and I still love crispy skin. This chicken recipe tastes much better and is much healthier.

It provides my taste buds with just the right seasonings and crispness--very juicy also.

Ingredients:

- 4 bone-in, skin-on, free-range chicken thighs

Skin-side seasoning:

- 1 teaspoon Kosher salt
- 1-2 tablespoons grass-fed butter (example: unsalted Kerrygold) or ghee

Meat-side seasoning:

- 1 tablespoon garlic powder
- 2 teaspoons dried oregano
- 1 teaspoon red pepper flakes
- 1 teaspoon sea salt

Preparation:

- Dry chicken with a paper towel.
- Cut out the bone, staying as close to the bone as possible. Don't cut off the skin. The skin makes the dish Yummy!
- Flatten the chicken with a meat pounder or just use your fist to pound it flat (That's how I take out my aggression.)
- Turn the chicken skin-side-up, and sprinkle Kosher salt on the skin (try to get the skin salted evenly).
- Heat a large skillet over medium high heat, and then melt the butter or ghee hot enough so that a sprinkle of water will splatter. Place four chicken thighs skin-side down in the skillet.
- Sprinkle the "meat seasoning" on the meat side.
- Cook the skin side until crispy and golden brown (around 7-10 minutes), You will need to have a splatter guard because the hot fat will splatter!
- Turn over the thighs and cook the meat side for 2-3 more minutes to thoroughly cook.

Consider using the remaining fat in the skillet to sauté some leafy green veggies to go along with this dish.

Crispy Salmon Filets

Wild-caught, Pacific salmon is one of my favorite fish. Salmon is loaded with healthy nutrients. This recipe is easy to make and keeps the skin crispy. It should be a real crowd pleaser, but check for small bones that may still be in the fillets. Since you will be placing the filets in hot butter fat, there will be splatter. A splatter guard over the pan is a great way to protect you from popping hot butter.

Ingredients:

- 2 (5-7-ounce) salmon fillets (be sure to check for bones; some are always there!)
- 1-2 tablespoons ghee or grass-fed butter
- Himalayan sea salt and freshly ground pepper to taste
- Zest of 1/2 lemon and squeeze of lemon juice

Preparation:

- Bring the salmon filets to room temperature and dry with paper towels.
- Generously salt and pepper both sides of the salmon filets.
- Heat a saucepan to medium high heat.
- Place ghee or butter and allow it to get hot (a sprinkle of water will splatter).
- Place the salmon filets in the pan, skin-side down.
- Cook for 4 minutes (skins will become crisp).
- Flip the filets, and cook for another 1 minute.
- Add squeeze of lemon and zest of lemon.
- Take the filets out of the pan and place on serving plate-- skin side up to keep crisp.
- Serve hot

Crispy Spiced Chicken Livers

Organ meats are nutrient dense and should be on everyone's menu at least once or twice a week. Liver is one of the best. This recipe takes liver to a crispy level that may be tastier for those who have not yet acquired the taste for other liver recipes.

Since you will be cooking in hot coconut oil, use a splatter screen to prevent dangerous oil splatter.

Ingredients:

- 2 cups whole raw almonds
- 1 tablespoon garlic powder
- 2 teaspoons dried oregano
- 1 teaspoon Himalayan salt
- 1/2 teaspoon red pepper flakes
- 1 pound pastured chicken livers, separated and patted dry
- 2 large eggs, beaten
- 6 Tablespoons virgin coconut oil

Preparation:

- Place almonds in food processor; pulse until ground into meal (don't over process or it will turn to almond butter); add garlic, oregano, salt, and pepper flakes and continue to pulse until mixed well. Place in separate bowl.
- Separate livers in half and dry thoroughly with paper towels.
- Beat eggs in separate bowl.
- Individually, dip each liver into beaten egg and then into seasoned almond meal.
- Place all coated livers on large plate and refrigerate to set coating (approximately 1/2 hour).
- Heat large non-stick frying pan over medium high heat and add coconut oil; heat oil until hot (sprinkle water on top of hot oil; if it splatters, it is hot enough).
- With tongs, place livers individually into hot oil (you will need a splatter screen)
- Cook, undisturbed, for 3 minutes on first side.
- Flip and cook an additional 2 minutes on the other side. They should be medium rare.
- Remove and serve

Curry Chicken-Thigh Salad

You can make the **Crispy Italian-spice Chicken Thighs**, and move right into this recipe to make the salad. The chicken tastes great; this salad recipe makes it even better--creaminess from the avocados and sweetness from the fruit.

Ingredients:

- 2 ripe avocados
- 4 crispy chicken thighs (previously made)
- 1 Tbs organic curry powder
- Sea salt and pepper
- 1/2 cup organic blueberries, other berries, or other dark-colored fruit

Preparation:

- Cut up avocados into small chunks; place into bowl; and mash into a paste.
- Cut up chicken thighs into bite-size pieces, place in bowl, and mix well
- Sprinkle curry powder; salt and pepper to taste and mix
- Add blueberries or other berries or other dark-colored fruit, and continue to mix.
- Serve as is or scoop into a bed of Romaine lettuce or butter lettuce

Dry Ribs in Slow Cooker

I love ribs--dry, spicy, fall-apart, melt-in-your-mouth ribs. But, I don't want the carbs from sugar or other unnatural ingredients that are frequently in commercial rubs. So, here is a recipe that offers everything I want from my ribs. See if this works for you.

Ingredients:

- 4-5 pounds of pastured pork ribs
- 1-2 large onions sliced thickly to cover bottom of slow cooker
- 2 tablespoons of coarse Kosher salt

- 1 tablespoon of cumin
- 1 tablespoon of fresh cracked pepper
- 1 1/2 tablespoons of dried oregano
- 1/2 tablespoon of chili powder
- 1 tablespoon of cinnamon
- 1 teaspoon of cayenne pepper

Preparation:

- Mix all spices together in a small bowl.
- Cut onions into thick slices and place them along the bottom of slow cooker. These will keep the ribs elevated off the bottom of the pot and away from drippings.
- Use paper towels to dry ribs.
- Generously apply dry rub to all surfaces of the ribs, and use up all rub mixture.
- Place ribs on top of onion layer with the "meat side" up.
- Set slow cooker on low, and cook for 8-10 hours.

French Onion Oxtail Stew in Slow Cooker

This is a super hearty and healthy dish[248], which I have tweaked to my liking. It has become one of my favorite dinners. Oxtails are rich in nutrients such as glucosamine, chondroitin, magnesium, glycine, and phosphorus, which help form bone cells, connective tissue, and collagen. Along with the bone broth as a base, you can see how healthy this stew is for joint and bone health.

This stew is especially delicious when it is placed on a bed of cauliflower mash. My cauliflower mash recipe is listed in this chapter.

Ingredients:

- 2 Tbs ghee (or butter) from grass-fed cows to brown oxtails
- 3 lbs. of cut-up oxtails
- Salt and pepper for oxtails
- 4 cloves garlic, chopped

- 1 tsp thyme
- 1/2 cup red wine
- 3 cups homemade bone broth
- 4 Tbs ghee (or butter) from grass-fed cows to caramelize onions
- 4 large sweet onions, peeled and thinly sliced
- Salt and pepper to taste (optional--red pepper flakes to taste)

Preparation:

- In a heavy skillet, heat ghee or butter over high heat.
- Season the oxtails liberally with salt and pepper
- Place oxtails in hot fat and brown on all sides
- Reduce heat to medium and add garlic
- Continue cooking for another minute or so to softly cook garlic
- Transfer oxtails and garlic to slow cooker
- Add wine, bone broth, and thyme to slow cooker and cook on low for 8 hours
- Before oxtails are done, add remaining ghee or butter to heavy covered skillet on medium-low heat
- Add onion to skillet, cover, and cook for about 15 minutes until onions are soft
- Remove cover and raise heat to medium stirring frequently, and cook until caramelized - onions will turn a deep golden color which may take an hour or so
- Once the oxtails are done in the slow cooker, remove oxtails with tongs and transfer to a large plate to cool
- Remove meat and gristle from bones and discard bones--I remove the meat and gristle with my fingers so I can feel for the inevitable small bones that could remain in the meat
- Transfer meat, gristle, and the remaining liquid from the slow cooker to the skillet containing the onions
- Continue on medium heat for 30-60 minutes to reduce liquid to thicken stew

- Salt and pepper to taste (optional: add red pepper flakes for heat)
- For a great meal, serve over cauliflower mash--unbelievable and healthy

French Onion Soup - Almost

The first time I had French Onion Soup was when my wife and I were in Montreal in the 1970s. What a delight! (That's when we had our first Crepe Suzettes--definitely way before my Primal education.) After returning from our vacation in Canada, we searched for the best French Onion Soup recipe. We found it in Julia Child's cookbook[249]. When I look at the ingredients now, they are not completely Paleo. So, I have tweaked the recipe and added some new stuff that I present below. Unfortunately, if you were looking for croutons, they aren't there.

Ingredients:

- 2 Lbs. sweet onions, thinly sliced
- 4 Tbs. butter or ghee
- 1 Tsp. salt
- 1 Tsp. turmeric
- 3 Tbs. arrowroot powder
- 6 Cups bone broth
- 1/2 Cup dry white wine
- Optional: raw mozzarella cheese as topping if you are eating raw dairy

Preparation:

- Slice onions thinly (I use a mandolin with the protection shield!)
- Heat butter or ghee in large covered skillet on medium-low heat
- Add onions and cook covered until onions have softened (about 15-20 minutes)

- Uncover, add salt and turmeric (turmeric stains everything!) and increase heat to medium-high and continue to cook until most of the liquid evaporates and the onions begin to brown slightly, which will take 45-60 minutes. Stir frequently.
- Add arrowroot powder stirring continuously to mix thoroughly
- Remove from heat and place onions in Dutch oven
- Deglaze skillet with white wine and add to Dutch oven
- Add bone broth to Dutch oven and bring to boil
- Simmer for 30-40 minutes
- Salt and pepper to taste
- Add raw mozzarella cheese when serving if you are eating raw dairy

Gumbo in Slow Cooker

Slow cookers make it so easy. My wife and I created this recipe, tried it, and fell in love with it. I think the combination of Shitake and Porcini mushrooms makes this dish so unusual. Use it as a side veggie dish or add protein such as shrimp and sausage to make a meal. Note that there is no extra water in this recipe, so it is thick and filling.

Ingredients:
- 6-quart Slow Cooker
- 4 Tbs grass-fed butter or ghee
- 1 sweet onion chopped
- 1/2 head of cabbage coarsely chopped or shredded
- 5 cloves garlic chopped
- 3 cups okra (sliced into 1/4 inch discs)
- 1 cup Shitake mushroom caps chopped
- 1 cup Porcini mushrooms chopped (At my local Costco, I found dried Porcini mushrooms that I reconstituted in warm water)
- 2 cans diced and fire roasted organic tomatoes with organic green chilies (14.5 oz. cans)

- Salt and pepper to taste
- Optional ingredients: fresh cooked shrimp; sliced, warmed organic Kielbasa sausage; etc.

Preparation:

- Place all ingredients except salt and pepper in slow cooker
- Cook on low heat for 6 hours
- Salt and pepper to taste and continue cooking on low if necessary for another 2 hours
- Serve hot (store remaining gumbo in containers to freeze for later use)
- Add extra ingredients such as shrimp, Kielbasa sausage, etc. to make a meal

Kale Chips

Nothing beats the slightly salty taste and crunchy texture of this simple snack. It's not a potato chip; it's a kale chip--very healthy and loaded with nutrients. Here is a simple recipe that can be made quickly. You can take this basic recipe and add other spices as you desire. Be creative. Cayenne pepper is a good choice for those who like a bit of heat. Some people like to prepare kale chips in an oven, and others like to use a dehydrator. This recipe is for the oven.

Ingredients:

- 1 bunch kale
- 2 Tablespoons coconut oil, melted
- 1 Tablespoon lemon juice
- Sea salt and freshly ground black pepper to taste

Preparation:

- Preheat oven to 300° F.
- Wash kale and dry as much as possible.
- Tear leaves off stems, and cut leaves into approximately 2-3 inch pieces.
- Place the kale in a bowl and drizzle with oil.

- Add salt and pepper to taste.
- Add lemon juice and disperse well.
- Place kale in a single layer on a baking sheet and place in oven for about 30 minutes, until crispy. Check on the chips every 10 minutes and toss them to make sure none of them overcook.
- Correct seasonings as necessary.

Kickin' Leafy Green Salad

You need to eat non-starchy veggies at every meal. A big salad serves the purpose. I am sure you have taken a bag of organic, prewashed greens, thrown them into a bowl, put some salt and pepper and olive oil on them and called it a salad. Yes, that is a salad. But, here is a kickin' salad. Simple, green, healthy, and with some heat.

Ingredients:

- 1 9-oz bag of ready-to-eat, organic romaine lettuce (any leafy greens would do)
- 1/4 tsp Himalayan salt
- 1/4 tsp red pepper flakes
- 1/2 tsp dried oregano spice
- 1 tsp garlic powder
- 1 can anchovies in extra virgin olive oil
- 1 avocado
- Extra virgin olive oil to taste

Preparation:

- Place greens in a big mixing bowl
- Combine salt, red pepper flakes, oregano, and garlic powder in small bowl
- Sprinkle mixture on greens and mix thoroughly
- Cut up anchovies into small pieces and add to greens along with its own olive oil and toss
- Cut up avocado into thin slices and add to greens and toss
- Add enough olive oil to taste and toss thoroughly

- You will be amazed by the KICK

Meatloaf Wrapped in Bacon in Slow Cooker

Meatloaf has always been a staple, quick meal in my home while growing up. Of course, the traditional meatloaf had bread and other ingredients that were not anything that resembled a Paleo compatible dish. Here is a recipe that not only is Paleo, but also includes organ meat--heart. There is a slightly spicy topping that tingles the palate, and you could add more red pepper flakes if you want more heat. The slow cooker and the addition of shiitake mushrooms keep the loaf moist and create a good amount of juice in the bottom of the pot. The juice is great to spoon over the meatloaf slices. Also, the meatloaf freezes well for later. By the way, bacon makes everything better!

Ingredients for Loaf:

- 1 lb grass fed/finished beef, ground
- 1 lb grass fed/finished beef heart, ground
- 3 cups shiitake mushroom caps, coarsely chopped
- 1 onion, chopped
- 5 garlic cloves, chopped
- 1 Tbs dried oregano
- 2 tsp sea salt
- 1 tsp pepper
- 2 large eggs, lightly beaten
- 1/2 lb pastured bacon (about 6 slices)

Ingredients for Topping:

- 4 Tbs tomato paste
- 2 tsp Dijon mustard
- 1/4 tsp red pepper flakes

Preparation:

- Combine all ingredients for meatloaf **except bacon** in large bowl and mix thoroughly
- Shape into an oval loaf in pot of 3-quart slow cooker

- Lay bacon strips side-to-side over loaf and tuck ends under loaf to maintain shape of loaf
- Combine ingredients for topping in small bowl and mix thoroughly
- Spread topping over top of bacon strips to cover completely
- Cover and cook on High for 1 hour; then cook on Low for 3 hours
- Remove from slow cooker and slice. Spoon the left over juice from the bottom of the pot over the meatloaf slices for more flavor and moisture

Mushroom and Seaweed Soup

This is an extremely healthy soup. It incorporates the many benefits of bone broth and the unique combination of the trace minerals and micronutrients found in a variety of seaweeds as well as the health benefits from mushrooms, onions, garlic, and fresh ginger. Some of the seaweeds and mushrooms you might find in the store or online dried, which will need to be reconstituted before using the suggested measurements below. You can experiment with the quantity of seaweeds and mushrooms to satisfy your individual taste.

TIP: The best way to grate ginger is to freeze an inch and then grate it while frozen. Easy!

Ingredients:
- 10-15 shiitake mushroom caps, quartered
- 10-15 porcini mushrooms, chopped
- 1/2 cup kelp seaweed, chopped
- 1/2 cup wakame seaweed, chopped
- 2 tablespoons coconut oil
- 1 medium sweet onion, quartered and sliced thin
- 3 cloves garlic, minced
- 6-8 cups warm bone broth
- 1-2 tablespoons minced fresh ginger

- 3-4 tablespoons coconut aminos
- 1 tablespoon rice wine vinegar
- 1/4 tsp red pepper flakes (optional)
- 1-2 teaspoons maple syrup--grade B (optional)
- Sea salt and freshly ground black pepper, to taste

Preparation:

- In a medium bowl, containing 2 cups lukewarm water, place the mushrooms and seaweed, then set aside for 20 minutes. Once the mushrooms and seaweed are soft, thoroughly rinse, strain, chop, and set aside.
- In a large pot, heat the oil over low heat and cook the onion and garlic until soft.
- Add in the bone broth, ginger, coconut aminos, vinegar, red pepper flakes, and the mushrooms and seaweed.
- Raise heat and bring mixture to a boil; then reduce to a simmer.
- Salt and pepper to taste
- Then simmer for 10 minutes.
- Remove from the heat, stir in maple syrup, and serve. Refrigerate or freeze leftovers for another day. Only reheat on the stove; a microwave can destroy nutrients.

No-Oat Oatmeal

I used to enjoy oatmeal in the morning--warm, nutty, yummy. Now I have a healthy Paleo substitute for an occasional splurge. Remember, the dates and any fruit toppings add fructose.

Ingredients:

- 1 cup of raw pumpkin seeds
- 1/2 cup of milled flax seeds
- 1/2 cup of macadamia nuts
- 6-8 pitted dates
- 1/2 Teaspoon of sea salt
- 1/2 Teaspoon vanilla

- Organic unsweetened coconut milk
- Optional: coconut cream; cinnamon; fresh berries, sliced banana

Preparation:

- Place the seeds, nuts, dates, sea salt and vanilla in food processor or blender and process for 2 minutes until you have a rough chopped mixture.
- Place the mixture in a glass jar to store in fridge.
- Take 1/2 cup of the mixture and 1 cup of coconut milk (more or less according to desired consistency) and place in a medium-size pan on stove.
- Bring to a boil and let simmer for 10 minutes.
- Optional: add coconut cream and/or fruit and/or cinnamon if desired

Plantain Pancakes

Pancakes were one of my favorite foods for breakfast before embracing a Primal Lifestyle. But, pancakes are made with wheat flour. There are coconut flour and almond flour recipes that avoid wheat flour, but they never had the taste and texture of real, chewy, soft pancakes. This recipe changed everything for me when I discovered delicious pancakes--the Paleo way! Try them, and judge for yourself. I have changed the original ingredients that I found on the Internet[250] to satisfy my tastes.

Ingredients:

- 2 large green plantains (about 2 cups pureed)
- 4 free-range eggs
- 4 Teaspoons of vanilla (more or less based on taste)
- 3 Tablespoons of extra virgin coconut oil
- 1/4 Teaspoon of sea salt
- 1/2 Teaspoon of baking soda
- Additional coconut oil for cooking

Preparation:

- Peel plantains. (It is easier to cut them lengthwise and then cut each section in half; then separate the peel from the meat of the plantain with your fingers.)
- Place plantain pieces into your food processor or powerful blender. (Vitamix or NutriBullet Rx.)
- Add the rest of the ingredients to the food processor or blender and process until it forms a smooth batter (about 1-2 minutes).
- Heat 1 Tablespoon of coconut oil in frying pan over medium-high heat. Pour the batter into the frying pan until your pancake is the desired size.
- Cook like a regular pancake. After 2-3 minutes, the top will form little bubbles just like a regular pancake. Flip it and cook the other side for another minute or so until done.
- Repeat until the batter runs out. Add a little coconut oil to the pan as needed.
- Top with butter, or honey, or grade B maple syrup, or whatever makes you happy!

Roasted Brussels Sprouts and Bacon

Is there a vegetable you or your family doesn't like even though you know that this veggie is healthy? My secret for getting just about anyone to love his or her "hated vegetable" is to cook some bacon with it. I think that anything is better if it is mixed with bacon. You might want to try chopped bacon bits on top of my custard dessert. Oh well, this is just me, but don't dismiss the idea until you've tried it.

I am only speaking about pastured bacon with no chemicals or artificial additives. Not the typical bacon you get at the grocery store.

Ingredients:

- 1 lb of bacon, pastured

- 2 lbs. of Brussels sprouts, fresh or frozen raw
- Salt and pepper to taste

Preparation:

- Heat saucepan to medium high heat
- Cut the bacon into small chunks and cook bacon until crispy (you should use a splatter screen to prevent oil splatter)
- Wash and cut Brussels sprouts in half and pat dry with paper towels as best as possible (if frozen, thaw completely and dry as best as possible)
- When the bacon is cooked, remove the bacon and put into a separate bowl
- Place the Brussels sprouts into the sauté pan with the bacon fat and cook over medium heat until Brussels sprouts are nicely browned.
- Add the bacon back to the pan and mix well.
- Salt and pepper to taste, and serve warm.

Roasted Cabbage Strips

Cabbage is a cruciferous vegetable and an excellent source of vitamin C, vitamin K, vitamin B6, folate and soluble fiber. Also, the phytochemicals in cabbage may stimulate the production of detoxifying enzymes and may have protective effects against colon cancer. The darker the color of the cabbage, the more phytochemicals present.

Here is a tasty way to serve and eat cabbage. The kelp granules add trace minerals and iodine, which are lacking in many prepared dishes. The recipe is easy and quick to prepare, but it will take 40 minutes or so in the oven. Give it a try.

Ingredients:

- 1 (approx. 2lb) head of organic purple cabbage (or any color), cut into 1" slices and then cut into 1-2" strips
- 1 Tsp Kelp granules
- 1 Tbs Garlic powder

- Himalayan salt taste
- Freshly ground black pepper
- 2 Tbs ghee or liquefied coconut oil

Preparation:

- Preheat oven to 400°F, and place parchment paper on baking sheet
- Place cut-up cabbage into large mixing bowl
- Add kelp, garlic, salt, and pepper to cabbage and toss
- Add ghee or liquefied coconut oil to cabbage and toss until well mixed
- Lay cabbage onto parchment paper, and place baking sheet in oven
- Roast on the middle rack for 20 minutes.
- Stir cabbage pieces and roast for an additional 20 minutes until edges become brown.
- Serve hot. Enjoy.

Option: Consider adding a leftover protein into the finished cabbage. For example, I had leftover chicken liver and onions from a previous dinner. I added them to the cabbage after I removed the cabbage from the oven. Surprisingly good!

Sardines for Sardine-Haters

Sardines are so healthy. One 4.375-ounce can of wild caught sardines with skin and bones contains about 310mg of EPA and 685mg of DHA omega-3 fatty acids. Also, a can contains ample amounts of vitamins B12 and D as well as selenium and coenzyme Q10. Ounce for ounce sardines contain more calcium and phosphorus than milk, more iron than spinach, more potassium than bananas, and as much protein as steak. But, most of my contemporaries say they don't eat sardines. Here is a simple way to serve sardines. Many sardine-haters would agree they aren't so bad when served this way. Try it. Who knows, you may become a sardine-lover.

Ingredients:

- 1 4.375-ounce can of wild caught pacific sardines with skin and bones (ex. Wild Planet, which is BPA free. They also package white anchovies, which has 4 times the amount of EPA that is in its can of sardines.)
- 1 large bell pepper, cut in half with seeds removed
- 1/2 fresh lime
- About 1/4 cup of fresh or thawed fruit (ex: blueberries, dark cherries, or strawberries)
- About 1/4 cup chopped nuts (ex: cashews, pistachios, almonds, or macadamia)
- Sprinkle of kelp granules for taste as well as trace minerals (ex: Maine Coast Sea Seasonings)
- Salt and pepper to taste

Preparation:

- Place both halves of a bell pepper on a plate
- Open the sardine can and drain liquid
- Place sardines into the open cavity of each pepper
- Squeeze fresh lime juice over sardines
- Top with fruit and nuts
- Sprinkle with kelp granules
- Add salt and pepper to taste
- Eat with your fingers or with knife and fork (more dainty)

Sautéed Super Greens

Leafy greens should be included with every meal. They are nutrient-dense and support healthy cells and their mitochondria. They can be eaten raw, or in smoothies, or steamed, or sautéed. There are amazing taste sensations and powerful nutrients in my Sautéed Super Greens aside from the greens themselves: heat from red pepper flakes, a bite from ginger, sweet from grade B maple syrup, acid from lemon juice, as well as nutrients from turmeric, onions, garlic, shitakes, and kelp. Love the turmeric, but be aware that it stains everything!

Ingredients:

- 4 Tbs ghee or grass-fed butter
- 1 sweet onion, chopped
- 5 cloves garlic, chopped
- 1 Tbs ginger, freshly grated
- 1 Tbs turmeric
- 1 Tsp red pepper flakes
- 1 Tsp kelp granules
- Salt and pepper to taste
- 2 cups shitake mushroom caps (cut into small pieces--not chopped)
- 4 cups cut and washed leafy greens (I like a mix of kale, spinach, and Swiss chard--but whatever you like will work)
- Freshly squeezed lemon juice
- 1 Tsp maple syrup (Grade B)

Preparation:

- Heat saucepan to medium heat
- Place ghee or butter and pan
- Add onions and garlic, and cook covered until soft (about 10 minutes)
- Add ginger, turmeric, red pepper flakes, and kelp granules; mix well
- Add salt and pepper to taste
- Add shitake mushrooms; cover; and cook until soft (about 5 minutes)
- Add leafy greens and additional salt and pepper to taste; sauté
- As soon as leafy greens begin to wilt, remove from heat and add squeeze of lemon juice and maple syrup
- Stir and let the flavors disperse
- Salt and pepper to taste if necessary
- Serve hot

Shepherd's Pie

I first had shepherd's pie at an Irish restaurant when I was a kid. As I remember, it was so good and so different from anything I ever had up to that point. Every now and then my wife and I would find it on the menu at a restaurant, and it was still a delight. Now, I have created a Paleo rendition.

Ingredients:

- 1 lb ground beef or lamb
- 1 large sweet onion chopped
- 3 cloves garlic chopped finely
- 1 Tbs rosemary
- 1 Tbs thyme
- 2 tsp paprika (and additional for sprinkling on Cauliflower Mash)
- 1 4-oz package of shitake mushrooms (only caps chopped and discard stems)
- 2 heaping Tbs organic tomato paste
- salt and pepper to taste
- 1 Tbs fat for pan (coconut oil or healthy fat of choice)

Preparation:

- Preheat over 350° F
- Mix all ingredients in bowl
- Heat oil in pan and place all ingredients to brown for 5 minutes
- Start Cauliflower Mash (see recipe in this section)
- Place meat and ingredients in 9 x 13 casserole dish and spread Cauliflower Mash over top and then sprinkle paprika on top
- Cook in oven for 40 minutes

Shrimp over Spaghetti Squash

Spaghetti squash is not a substitute for pasta. Spaghetti squash is significantly healthier than pasta and actually can be as satisfying as pasta. This is a great recipe, and the shrimp are succulent--just as they were meant to be eaten. There are 4 parts to this recipe: cutting, cooking, and shredding the squash; preparing the garlic butter sauce; cooking the perfect shrimp; and putting them all together.

Ingredients:

- 1 medium spaghetti squash
- Ghee or grass-fed butter for squash
- Salt and pepper for squash
- 4 Tbs ghee or grass-fed butter for garlic butter sauce
- 5 garlic cloves, chopped for garlic butter sauce
- Salt and pepper for garlic butter sauce
- 2 Tbs Old Bay Seasoning for shrimp
- 1 lb raw shrimp, peeled and deveined
- Optional garnishes: parsley, kelp granules, fresh lemon or lime squeeze

Preparation:

- Cut, cook, and shred the spaghetti squash (see #1 below)
- Prepare garlic/butter sauce (see #2 below)
- Cook perfect shrimp (see #3 below)
- Put them all together and enjoy (see #4 below)

#1 Cut, Cook, and Shred Squash:

You must cut the raw spaghetti squash in half lengthwise with a sharp, sturdy chef's knife. The outer shell is hard and the squash rolls around easily!

Start by cutting off the stem with a sharp knife. Cut a groove in the surface about 1/2 inch deep from end to end lengthwise on one side using a paring knife. Next, hold one end of the squash with one hand. With your other hand, place your heavy-duty chef's knife in the middle of the squash in the groove with the blade facing AWAY from the hand holding the squash. Press straight down with your chef's knife until the tip of the blade meets the other side. Then, pull the knife down (away from your hand that is holding the other end) along the groove, cutting one side in half.

Repeat the process to cut through the other half of the squash with the blade facing AWAY from the hand holding the squash on the opposite end.

Separate the halves and scoop the seeds out with a spoon. Discard the seeds. Place each half (shell side down) in a casserole dish and brush ghee on each surface. Salt and pepper to taste. **Cover** the casserole dish and place in the microwave for 5 minutes on high. Check with a fork to see if the flesh of the squash is soft. If not, place in the microwave covered for an additional 2 minutes and check again. Repeat until the flesh is soft. Then let cool covered for about 15 minutes. After it has cooled so you can handle it, use a fork to gently scrape the flesh of the squash to shred it into strands that actually look similar to spaghetti. Set aside in the dish from which you will serve, and cover until ready to use.

#2 Prepare Garlic Butter Sauce

Place ghee or butter in a saucepan and warm. Add chopped garlic and cook on low heat until garlic is soft. Salt and pepper to taste. Keep saucepan covered until ready to use.

#3 Cook Perfect Shrimp

Place about 4-cups of water in a pot with 2 Tbs of Old Bay Seasoning and bring to a boil. Then add 1-pound raw shrimp just until the flesh becomes opaque (no more than 1-2 minutes). Immediately remove from stove and pour through a strainer disposing of the liquid.

#4 Put Them All Together

Add shrimp to shredded spaghetti squash. Drizzle with the garlic butter sauce. Serve and enjoy. You can garnish with parsley and kelp granules. Also, you could drizzle some fresh lemon or lime juice over the shrimp.

Shrimp Sautéed with Pork Belly and Herbs

Everything is better with bacon. But, this is not really bacon. It's the pork belly before it became bacon. It's really good, and you have control over the seasoning. The sauce is optional as well as the greens. The remaining hot fat from the pork belly is great for sautéing, so I would use it for some sautéed veggies on the side.

Ingredients:

Shrimp

- 1 pound large wild-caught shrimp, shelled and deveined
- 1/2 teaspoon garlic powder
- 1 teaspoon parsley
- 1 teaspoon finely chopped rosemary
- salt and pepper to taste

Pork Belly (unseasoned bacon)

- 1 pound sliced pastured pork belly, cut into 2 inch bits
- 1/2 teaspoon garlic powder
- 1 teaspoon parsley
- 1 teaspoon finely chopped rosemary
- salt and pepper to taste

Sauce (optional)

- 2 teaspoons fresh lemon juice
- 2 tablespoons ghee or unsalted grass-fed butter
- 1 teaspoon dulse flakes

Salad Greens (optional)

Vegetables for sautéing (optional)

Preparation:

- In a medium bowl, toss shrimp, garlic, rosemary, parsley, salt and pepper. Set aside to marinate at room temperature for 30 minutes. In a different bowl, do the same for the pork belly.
- Place pork belly in a large skillet, and place over medium-high heat. Cook, stirring occasionally, until almost all the

259

fat is rendered, and the pork belly is browned, 6 to 7 minutes. Remove pork belly.

- Add the shrimp to pork belly grease; sauté, turning frequently, until the shrimp are opaque and just cooked through, about 1-2 minutes. DO NOT OVERCOOK! Remove shrimp.
- Place shrimp and pork belly onto plate
- If desired, place shrimp and pork belly over fresh greens.
- If desired, melt ghee or butter and add lemon juice. Salt and pepper to taste. Pour over shrimp and pork belly. Sprinkle dulse over shrimp and pork belly.
- If desired, sauté vegetables in pork belly grease; salt and pepper to taste. Plate as a side dish.

Sue's Reuben Salad

Here's a twist. My wife, Sue, came up with this idea, and it's really good. I'm sure you have been introduced to The Reuben Sandwich somewhere along your way. It is a popular Deli delight. Sue created this Paleo answer to the taste of a Reuben--of course without the unhealthy meat, the bread or the unhealthy dressing. Give it a try; you might be pleasantly surprised--we were! Be aware that there is real raw cheese in this dish.

Ingredients:

- 4-cups spring mix (or any mixed greens)
- 1-2 Tbs extra virgin olive oil
- Himalayan sea salt, ground pepper to taste
- 1 lb Sautéed pastured-pork breakfast sausage broken up into crumbles
- 1/2-cup Bubbies' Sauerkraut (or any live-culture sauerkraut)
- 1/2-cup raw Swiss cheese
- 1 Tbs oregano
- Himalayan sea salt, ground pepper to add to oregano topping

Preparation:

- Add olive oil, salt, and pepper to salad and toss--taste
- Place salad into casserole bowl that is oven proof
- Place sautéed breakfast sausage on top of salad
- Place sauerkraut on top of sausage crumbles
- Place cheese on top of sauerkraut
- Sprinkle oregano, salt and pepper on top of cheese
- Set oven to broil and place dish in oven 6 inches below broiler and allow cheese to melt (approx. 5-10 minutes)
- Serve

Thai Shrimp and Coconut Soup

I enjoy the flavor of coconut--not to mention shrimp. Thai inspired coconut soup hits the spot for me especially in the winter months. But for me, soup is good anytime--especially when the base is homemade bone broth.

For coconut soup, I like it to have a thicker consistency rather than a thin consistency. One way to accomplish this is to use only the cream in the coconut milk as I describe below. Also, you could continue to boil the liquid before adding the raw shrimp to reduce the liquid and thicken the soup further. I substitute the typical ingredient of fish sauce with a homemade concoction of mashed anchovies in coconut aminos.

Ingredients:

- 1 pound wild caught shrimp
- Coconut cream from 1 can (15.5 ounces) full-fat coconut milk
- 1 Tablespoon raw coconut aminos
- 1 2-oz can of anchovy fillets (drain oil)
- 2 cups bone broth
- 1 inch piece of ginger, peeled and grated
- 1 cup sliced shitake mushrooms
- 2 Tablespoons lime juice

- Salt and pepper to taste
- Cilantro for garnish (optional)

Preparation:

- Prepare the shrimp by peeling and deveining if not already done prior to purchase; dry shrimp with paper towel.
- Place can of coconut milk upside down into freezer for 5 minutes, which allows the cream to solidify on top and separate from the liquid on the bottom. Open other end, pour off liquid, and remove cream.
- Chop up anchovies and mix into coconut aminos in separate small mixing bowl
- In a pot over medium heat, combine anchovies mixed with aminos, coconut cream, bone broth, ginger, mushrooms, lime juice
- Bring to a boil (let boil for several minutes to reduce liquid if desired).
- Salt and pepper to taste
- Add shrimp, and cook until tender which will only be additional 1-2 minutes (do not overcook shrimp)
- Top with fresh chopped cilantro for garnish.

Tomatoes with Oil and Basil

Great taste and easy to prepare. I set them in a bowl for snacking or as a side dish with a meal.

Ingredients:

- 1 package of grape tomatoes
- 2 Tbs olive oil or macadamia oil
- 1/2 Tsp salt
- 1/2 Tsp pepper
- 1 Tbs fresh, chopped basil (1 Tsp if dried basil)

Preparation:

- Place tomatoes in bowl
- Add all ingredients and toss
- How is that for simplicity?

Wild Caught Salmon in Parchment

Salmon is very healthy, but make sure your salmon is not farm raised. Wild-caught Pacific Northwest salmon is my choice. This recipe allows the salmon to be especially moist because the parchment paper allows the steam to remain in the pouch. Make sure all the bones are removed. Even though it is a "fillet", I have always found at least one annoying bone. If you rub your finger along the flesh, you might feel the tip of an obscure bone. Use a tweezers to pull it out; it will be longer than you think.

You could easily embellish this simple recipe by adding other spices and possibly some ground nuts of your choice into the softened butter before placing it on top of the fillets before closing the pouch.

Ingredients:
- 2 (5-7-ounce) salmon fillets (be sure to check for bones; some are always there!)
- Himalayan sea salt and freshly ground pepper to taste
- Juice and zest of 1/2 lemon
- 1/2 tsp Herbs de Provence
- 2 tablespoons softened grass-fed butter

Preparation:
- Preheat the oven to 400° F.
- Sprinkle a little salt on the skin side of the salmon.
- Lay the fish, skin-side down, on individual sheets of parchment paper.
- Salt and pepper meat side to taste.
- Squeeze juice and sprinkle zest on fillets.
- Mix Herbs de Provence into the softened butter.
- Generously heap softened butter on top of the fillets.
- Fold the parchment paper into pouches. Your goal is to make a tightly sealed pouch in which the fish will steam.

- Place the parchment pouches on a baking sheet and slide them into the oven on the center rack.
- Bake for 10-11 minutes.
- When done, carefully unwrap the parchment paper. (The salmon may need more time to cook based on the thickness of the fillets.) Open carefully; the escaping steam will be very hot. Serve the fish with its own juices in their individual pouches or remove salmon and place on plates along with nutrient-dense green veggies prepared whatever way you desire.

Special Dishes

Burger, Fries, and a Soda

Before I got educated about primal nutrition and lifestyle, my go-to quick meal was usually a burger, fries, and a soda--a junk-food meal with little to no nutrition. Here's a healthier Paleo idea with no junk, lots of nutrients, and satisfying tastes and crunches.

In place of the burger, mix up some grass-fed/grass-finished ground beef with some salt, pepper, garlic, and any other spices you want. Form them into patties, and grill them or cook them on the stovetop like any hamburger. Wrap them with Romaine lettuce leaves, add a sauce such as mustard or organic tomato paste or my Healthier Mayo and *voila!* Your very own healthy Paleo burger.

In place of the soda, have a yummy, healthy, fermented Kombucha--a fermented ice tea that is loaded with fizz, flavor, and gut healthy probiotics and antioxidants. My favorite brand is GT's Organic Raw Kombucha®.

And to top it off, here are healthier, crunchy, salty fries--sweet potato fries. They are easy to make and satisfying.

There you have it: the go-to-junk-food meal in a Paleo-healthier form.

Sweet Potato Fries

Great-tasting fries, and healthier, too!

Ingredients:

- 2-3 small sweet potatoes with skins
- 4 tablespoons melted coconut oil
- Salt and pepper to taste

Preparation:

- Preheat oven to 400° F. Slice the sweet potatoes into thin French fry strips (cut into quarters and then into thin slices--a julienne slicer would make is easier).
- Place them in a large mixing bowl, and add oil to drench them.
- Sprinkle with sea salt and fresh black pepper.
- Toss until they are well coated.
- Place them in a single layer on a baking sheet lined with parchment paper, making sure they're not overlapping or touching.
- Place in the oven and bake for 20 minutes. Check continuously.
- You may need to bake another 5 to 10 minutes until tender, crisp, and golden; avoid burning.

Healthy Thanksgiving

Thanksgiving is a time for family and friends to get together for good food, good fun, and to give thanks for everything life has to offer. But, this is also a time for overindulgence of unhealthy treats. The main food offenders that cause a host of issues are processed foods made with grains and sugars. If you could eliminate these food products, your body would be so much better off, and your mouth would smile. Stuffing and dessert could be the most challenging, so I have focused on healthy solutions for both of these--a healthy stuffing on the side and a healthy pumpkin pie. YUM!

Healthy Stuffing on the Side

Stuffing is always a problem because of the grains and sugars that are part of the recipes. Here is a simple recipe for a healthy stuffing:

Ingredients:

- 4-5 small sweet potatoes, peeled and cut into 1/2 inch pieces
- 4 tablespoons coconut oil (warm to make liquid)
- salt & freshly ground pepper
- 4 celery stalks, thinly chopped
- 2 medium onions, chopped
- 4 cloves garlic, chopped
- 8 oz. country style ground pork sausage, crumbled (preferably pastured pork)
- 2 cups shiitake mushroom caps, roughly chopped
- 1/2 cup dry white wine
- 2 large eggs, beaten (preferably pastured eggs)
- 1/2 cup chicken bone broth (see my Bone Broth in Slow Cooker recipe)
- 4 pitted dates, finely chopped
- 3tablespoons chopped fresh sage
- 1/2 cup chopped pecan

Preparation:

- Preheat oven to 400° F. In large bowl, toss the sweet potatoes with 1-tablespoon coconut oil and sprinkle with 1/2-teaspoon salt and 1/4-teaspoon pepper. Place potatoes on baking sheet (lined with parchment paper) one layer thick and roast in oven until just tender, about 20 minutes.
- Meanwhile, heat 3-tablespoons coconut oil in a large skillet over medium heat. Add the celery, onions, garlic, and 1-teaspoon salt, and 1/4-teaspoon pepper. Cook, stirring occasionally, until vegetables are softened, about 10 to 12 minutes. Add the sausage and cook through until thoroughly browned.

- Add mushrooms and wine; cook until liquid evaporates, 2 to 4 minutes.
- Transfer the mixture to a large bowl along with the roasted sweet potatoes and let everything cool for 10 minutes or so. Turn oven down to 375° F.
- Add the beaten eggs, chicken stock, pecans, dates, and sage to the veggie/meat mixture and combine well. Use coconut oil to grease a 9-by-13-inch baking dish. Transfer the mixture to the prepared baking dish. Cover with aluminum foil and bake for 20 minutes. Remove the foil and bake until browned, 20 to 30 minutes more.

Healthy Pumpkin Pie

Refined sugars and flours are usually ingredients of every dessert. Here is a healthy Pumpkin Pie recipe without added flours or unnatural sugars.

Ingredients:

Crust

- 1 cup pecans
- 1/2 cup hazelnuts
- 4 tablespoons coconut oil (warmed to make liquid)
- 1/4 teaspoon sea salt
- extra coconut oil to grease pie pan

Filling

- 1 can organic pumpkin puree (usually 15 oz.)
- 2 eggs, beaten
- 1/2 cup local raw honey
- 1/2 cup organic coconut cream (Native Forest is a good brand)
- 2 teaspoon cinnamon
- 1/4 teaspoon ground cloves
- 1/4 teaspoon ground ginger

Preparation:

- Preheat your oven to 350° F.
- Grind nuts in a food processor into a flour consistency. Don't over process; it will turn into butter.
- In a bowl, create the crust mixture by mixing the processed nuts, coconut oil, and salt; then spread the mixture into a 9-inch glass pie pan greased with coconut oil and bake for 10 minutes.
- While the crust bakes, mix the filling ingredients together in a bowl.
- Add the filling evenly into the baked crust and bake for an additional 45 minutes.

Miscellaneous

Best Overall Seasoning

This is my go-to seasoning for everything when I want a little heat. I use it on salads, on eggs, on cooked veggies, on almost anything. Obviously, it's a matter of taste.

I make this and store it to use whenever I want.

Ingredients:

- 3 Tbs garlic powder
- 2 Tbs Oregano flakes
- 1 Tbs Himalayan salt
- 1 Tbs red pepper flakes

Preparation:

- Mix together and store in jar with a lid. What could be easier?

Bone Broth in Slow Cooker

Bone broth has been called the miracle drink. It is loaded with healing nutrients--some of which you only can get from homemade bone broth. Here are a few of the benefits:

- Helps heal and seal your gut, and promotes healthy digestion
- Inhibits infection caused by cold and flu viruses
- Fights inflammation
- Promotes strong, healthy bones
- Promotes healthy hair and nail growth

This is easy to make if you use the slow cooker. Once everything is in the pot and you turn it on, it will do its wonders.

Ingredients:

- 6-quart Slow Cooker
- 2-4 lbs. grass-fed/grass-finished beef bones and/or pastured chicken or pork bones and/or venison bones (ideally marrow, oxtail, knuckles, and feet bones from young animals)
- 4 Tbs apple cider vinegar (to help leach the minerals from the bones)
- 1 onion, roughly chopped
- 3 cloves garlic, roughly chopped
- 2 celery stalks, roughly chopped
- 2 carrots, roughly chopped
- 1 bunch fresh parsley
- Salt and pepper to taste

Preparation:

- Place bones in a crock-pot.
- Add apple cider vinegar
- Cover with water
- Cook at low temperature ideally for a total of 24-48 hours
- When 4 cooking-hours are left, add chopped vegetables (except parsley)
- 10 minutes before completion, add parsley
- Remove bones and vegetables with a large, slotted spoon
- Let cool down and strain remaining broth to collect all the liquid

- Portion out and use it as a drink or use it in recipes; salt and pepper to taste only the broth you will use now
- You must freeze whatever you will not use in the next 3-4 days to avoid possible bacterial growth. You can freeze broth in a Mason jar (leave air space for expansion or the glass could crack) or ice-cube trays. Flexible silicone baking trays also work well. When you reheat the bone broth, only do it in a saucepan (not in the microwave) to preserve nutrients.

Easy Ghee

I love ghee. It is delicious. No milk solids and all butter fat--full of fat-soluble vitamins only if you use grass-fed cow butter. Anyplace where you would use butter, you could substitute ghee. I also use it with my Bulletproof Coffee, which has been popularized by David Asprey. I have the recipe for my spiced version here in the recipe section.

Ingredients:

- 1 lb grass-fed butter (unsalted Kerrygold is a reliable brand)
- 16 oz Mason jar
- Funnel to place into Mason jar
- Natural Brown #4 size coffee filter (ex: Melita) or cheesecloth placed into funnel

Preparation:

- Begin to heat a saucepan on low heat
- Place butter in pan
- Butter will melt slowly and white foam will start to form on top
- As butter continues to heat, the white foam will start to precipitate into white particles that settle to the bottom (these are the milk solids), and the liquid (this will be the pure butter fat) will start bubbling (be aware of splatter)

- As the bubbling subsides, the white particles on the bottom will start to brown
- Pour liquid from saucepan into the funnel lined with the coffee filter (this liquid is very hot!)
- The golden liquid that collects in the Mason jar is pure, delicious, healthy butter fat. This is the ghee. The ghee does not have to be refrigerated; use for cooking or whatever suits you. Ghee is the perfect cooking oil. It is stable at temperatures to 500 degrees F.

Healthier Mayo

Look at the ingredients in the mayonnaise you purchase from the store--a lot of additives are pumped into the jar. Especially troublesome are the seed and vegetable oils that make up most of the mayo. These oils have high levels of omega-6 fatty acids, are overly processed and easily oxidized, and are very unstable in the body. Here is an easy-to-make and healthier mayo, which has become my family's go-to-mayo for all dressing, spreading, and cooking needs. I first learned how to make this from Melissa Joulwan's fantastic cookbook, *Well Fed.* [251] This is easily transformed into different dressings when you mix in various herbs and spices. Use your imagination.

Ingredients:
- 1 egg (pastured, free range) at room temperature
- ½ tsp dry mustard
- ½ tsp sea salt
- 1 ¼ cups light olive oil (also known as tasting olive oil)
- ½ lemon (juice squeezed and at room temperature)
- Stick Blender (ex: Cuisinart Hand Blender with 24 oz mixing beaker)

Preparation:
- Place whole egg, mustard, salt, and ¼ cup of oil in mixing beaker. Be sure that egg is at room temperature.

- Blend with Stick Blender until smooth.
- Add the remaining 1-cup of oil while continuously blending. The mixture will become thick and the consistency of mayo.
- Add lemon juice (be sure it is at room temperature) and continue to blend until completely incorporated into the mayo. (I have learned that if you add the lemon juice before this step, the mayo will have a looser consistency and will tend to separate later.)
- Refrigerate until needed. *Yum!*

Hollandaise Sauce

Hollandaise is one of those sauces to splurge on, perfect for a special brunch or a party with friends.

Emulsions are a type of mixtures where you force two liquids that normally wouldn't go together to mix. Mayo is another example of an emulsion. The key to an emulsion is to add the fat - the ghee in this case - very slowly while blending or whisking so the emulsion won't "break" or separate. Take your time. This is fun.

Ingredients:
- 1/2 cup melted ghee
- 2 egg yolks
- 1 Tablespoon lemon juice
- Pinch of salt
- Pinch of cayenne pepper or dash of hot sauce

Preparation:
- Gently melt the ghee on the stove. It should only be warm.
- Place the egg yolks, lemon juice, salt and cayenne pepper in the blender or Vitamix.
- Start the blender on low and run for about 30 seconds. Slowly drizzle the melted ghee into the blender through the hole in the lid. You must go slowly or the emulsion will separate and get soupy.

- Once all the ghee is added and the Hollandaise has thickened, you're done. Scrape it out and use on eggs, roasted veggies, a juicy steak...whatever your heart desires.
- This should keep for a couple days in the fridge though it will harden when it cools. Gently warm on the stove if desired. If you over heat it, the egg yolk will cook.

iv. Personal Forms

The next several pages consist of forms that I have my own patients complete prior to performing any treatment. I want to know their past medical history as well as their dental history and overall body concerns. This includes the foods they eat and why they want to make a change in their lifestyle. By reviewing the questions and providing your own answers, you may well learn something about yourself that you never knew before! And help your family learn about themselves, as well!

QUESTIONNAIRE

Date: _____

Name:_____
Male □ Female □

Age:_____ Weight:_____

Height:_____ Blood Pressure:_____

Current Medical Conditions (Be Specific):

Current Allergies (Be Specific):

Current Prescription Medications (Be Specific):

Current Supplements, Prebiotics, Probiotics, Herbs, Over-the-counter Medicines, etc. (Be Specific):

Understanding Your Mouth

Are you happy with your smile?
Yes □ No □

If no, what is not right?

Have you had treatments for gum disease?
Yes □ No □
If yes, what were the treatments?

Do your gums bleed?
Yes □ No □

Do you have swelling in your gums?
Yes □ No □

Are you having any pain in your mouth?
Yes □ No □
If yes, please explain.

Do you have gum disease now?
Yes □ No □
If yes, why do you think you have it?

Did anything change in your life when you first noticed your gum condition?
Yes □ No □ NA □
If yes, be specific:

Has anything made your gum problems better or worse?
Yes □ No □ NA □
If yes, be specific:

Do you have gum recession?
Yes □ No □
If yes, is it getting worse or staying the same?

Have your wisdom teeth been extracted?
Yes □ No □
If yes, which have been extracted?

Have you ever had mercury (silver colored) fillings?
Yes □ No □
If yes, do you still have these fillings?
Yes □ No □

How often do you brush your teeth?

How often do you floss?

If you have ever had dental braces, please explain.

Do you have sensitive teeth?
Yes □ No □
If yes, what makes them sensitive?

Do you have loose teeth?
Yes □ No □
If yes, be specific:

Do you have headaches in the morning?
Yes □ No □

Do you have jaw muscle soreness?
Yes □ No □

Do you have clicking or popping in your jaws?
Yes □ No □

Do you use any type of a bite guard?
Yes □ No □

Have you ever been treated for TMJ or jaw joint problems?
Yes □ No □
If yes, be specific:

Are you missing any teeth?
Yes □ No □
If yes, where are you missing teeth?

If you have missing teeth, have they been replaced with artificial teeth?
Yes □ No □
  If yes, how have they been replaced?

Understanding Your Body

If you had a magic wand and could eliminate three health/nutrition problems, what would they be?
  1.
  2.
  3.

What part or aspect of your body bugs you the most?

Have you ever had a nutrition consultation?
Yes □ No □
If yes, please describe:

What does "food" mean to you?

Have you made any changes in your eating habits because of your health?
Yes □ No □
If yes, please describe:

Do you currently follow a special diet or nutritional program?
Yes □ No □
If yes, please describe:

If you were going to change your diet, would you want to jump in and do it all at once, or would you want to take it slowly?

Do you avoid any particular foods?
Yes □ No □
If yes, please describe:

What percentage of the following meals do you eat out?
- Breakfast?
- Lunch?
- Dinner?

How much time passes between each meal you eat?

Do you have food cravings?
Yes □ No □
If yes, please describe:

Do you ever fast?
Yes □ No □
If yes, please describe:

What quenches your thirst during the day?

What are your personal challenges to eating well?

Do you personally go grocery shopping?
Yes □ No □
If no, who does?

Do you cook?
Yes □ No □
If no, who does?

Are you willing to learn new ways of cooking and buying food
Yes □ No □
If no, please explain:

What do you think would make the most positive difference in your overall health?

Please record the following measurements in centimeters with a tape measure:
- Waist circumference (the smallest circumference at or above your belly button):
- Hip circumference (the fullest circumference around your buttocks area):

Rate the following on a scale of 1 (not willing) to 5 (very willing)

In order to improve your health, how willing are you to:
- Significantly modify your diet: 1 2 3 4 5
- Modify your lifestyle (work, sleep, eating): 1 2 3 4 5
- Engage in regular exercise/physical activity: 1 2 3 4 5
- Have periodic lab tests to assess your progress: 1 2 3 4 5
- Keep a 3-day record of everything you eat and drink: 1 2 3 4 5

Do you exercise?
Yes □ No □
If yes, please describe:

Do you sleep well?
Yes □ No □
If no, please explain:

On average, how many hours of sleep do you get per night?

Do you use any type of tobacco?
Yes □ No □
If yes, what type tobacco, how much, and how often?

Do you use any type of alcohol?
Yes □ No □

If yes, what type of alcohol, how much, and how often?

Do you feel as if you have little energy?
Yes □ No □
If yes, please explain:

Do you have cold hands?
Yes □ No □

Do you have cold feet?
Yes □ No □

How many hours a week do you spend in the sun?

Of those hours in the sun, for how many of them are you covered with a sunscreen product?

Do you have "stomach issues"?
Yes □ No □
If yes, please describe:

Do you have generalized aches and pains?
Yes □ No □
If yes, please describe:

YOUR STORY

Date:_____

In your own words, explain WHY it is important for you to make a change in your life.

Three-Day Food Journal

It is important to keep an accurate record of your usual food and beverage intake. Complete the following "Food Journal" for three consecutive days including one weekend day.

Do not change your eating behavior at this time. The purpose of this food record is to analyze your present eating habits

Record information as soon as possible after the food has been consumed

Identify who you were eating with (spouse, family, friend, alone)

Describe all foods and beverages consumed as accurately and in as much detail as possible including estimated amounts.

Record the amount of each food or beverage consumed using standard measurements such as 8 ounces, 1 cup, 1 teaspoon, etc.

Include any added items, for example: tea with 1 teaspoon of honey, potato with 2 teaspoons butter, etc.

List all beverages and types, including water, coffee, tea, sports drinks, sodas/diet sodas, etc.

Comment on any noted emotional mood (happy, excited, depressed) or physical symptoms including hunger level, stress, bloating, fatigue, adverse reaction experienced, etc.

Include comments about eating habits and environment such as reasons for skipping a meal; when a meal was eaten at a restaurant, in a car, at a picnic, etc.

Explain any exercise or other type of physical activity you do each day and when you do them

Each day note all bowel movements, describe their consistency (regular, loose, firm, etc.), frequency, and any additional information

List supplements or medications including the amount and time you take them each day.

Day 1

Date: _____ Day of Week: _____

Meal:	Food and Beverages	Mood and/or Symptoms
Breakfast Time:		
Snack Time:		
Lunch Time:		
Snack Time:		
Dinner Time:		
Snack Time:		

Explain Any Exercise or Physical Activity

Bowel Movements

Time:
Description:

Time:
Description:

Time:
Description:

Day 2

Date: _____ Day of Week: _____

Meal:	Food and Beverages	Mood and/or Symptoms
Breakfast Time:		
Snack Time:		
Lunch Time:		
Snack Time:		
Dinner Time:		
Snack Time:		
Explain Any Exercise or Physical Activity		

Bowel Movements
Time: Description:
Time: Description:
Time: Description:

Day 3

Date: _____   Day of Week: _____

Meal:	Food and Beverages	Mood and/or Symptoms
Breakfast Time:		
Snack Time:		
Lunch Time:		
Snack Time:		
Dinner Time:		
Snack Time:		
Explain Any Exercise or Physical Activity		

Bowel Movements

Time:
Description:

Time:
Description:

Time:
Description:

INDEX

REFERENCES

[1] http://www.nidcr.nih.gov/DataStatistics/FindDataByTopic/Dental Caries/DentalCariesAdults20to64.htm

[2] http://www.nidcr.nih.gov/DataStatistics/FindDataByTopic/Dental Caries/DentalCariesSeniors65older.htm

[3] Li, Y; Lee. S; et al. Prevalence and severity of gingivitis in American adults. Am J Dent. 2010 Feb;23(1):9-13.

[4] Eke, P.I.; Dye, B.A.; Wei, L.; Thornton-Evans, G.O.; Genco, R.J. Prevalence of Periodontitis in Adults in the United States: 2009 and 2010. JDR. 2012:10, 914-920.

[5] http://www.perio.org/consumer/cdc-study.htm

[6] In gratitude to: Kripalu Nutrition Intensive (www.kripalu.org) and my various nutrition teachers (John Bagnulo, Kathie Swift, Annie Kay, Jennifer Young, Susan Lord, Lisa Nelson, Mel Sotos, Patrick Hanaway, Jay Lombard, Jim Gordon, Cindy Geyer, Jeanne Wallace, Coco Newton, Mark Hyman, Brenda Davis, Mark Sisson, and Chris Kresser) who have enlightened me on this journey to wellness. Also my son, Michael Danenberg (www.performance-therapy.com), an Active Release Technique Therapist and a strength training and nutrition coach for over 20 years who has encouraged me for many years to get my act together about nutrition and fitness training.

[7] Gurven, M; Kaplan, H. Longevity among hunter-gatherers: a cross-cultural examination. Population and Development Review. 2007:33(2), 321-365.

[8] Meyer, M; Fu, Q; et al. A mitochondrial genome sequence of a hominin from Sima de los Huesos. Nature. 2014, 1, 403-406.

[9] Adler, Christina J, et al. Sequencing ancient calcified dental plaque shows changes in oral microbiota with dietary shifts of the Neolithic and Industrial revolutions. Nature Genetics. 2013:45 450-455.

[10] Humphrey, L.T.; De Groote; I.; Morales, J.; Barton, N.; Collcutt, S.; Bronk Ramsey, C.; Bouzouggar, A. Earliest evidence for caries and exploitation of starchy plant foods in Pleistocene hunter-gatherers from Morocco. Proc Natl Acad Sci U S A 2014, 3, 954-9.

[11] Adler, Christina J, et al. Sequencing ancient calcified dental plaque shows changes in oral microbiota with dietary shifts of the Neolithic and Industrial revolutions. Nature Genetics. 2013:45 450-455.

[12] Ibid.

[13] Humphrey, L.T.; De Groote; I.; Morales, J.; Barton, N.; Collcutt, S.; Bronk Ramsey, C.; Bouzouggar, A. Earliest evidence for caries and exploitation of starchy plant foods in Pleistocene hunter-gatherers from Morocco. Proc Natl Acad Sci U S A 2014, 3, 954-9.

[14] Adler, Christina J, et al. Sequencing ancient calcified dental plaque shows changes in oral microbiota with dietary shifts of the Neolithic and Industrial revolutions. Nature Genetics. 2013:45 450-455.

[15] Hujoel, P. Dietary carbohydrates and dental systemic diseases. J Dent Res. 2009: 88(6), 490-502.

[16] Klaus, HD; Tam, ME. Oral health and the postcontact adaptive transition: a contextual reconstruction of diet in Morrope, Peru. Am J Phys Anthropol. 2010: 141(4), 594-609.

[17] Adler, Christina J, et al. Sequencing ancient calcified dental plaque shows changes in oral microbiota with dietary shifts of the Neolithic and Industrial revolutions. Nature Genetics. 2013:45 450-455.

[18] Spreadbury, Ian. Comparison with ancestral diets suggests dense acellular carbohydrates promote an inflammatory microbiota, and may be the primary dietary cause of leptin resistance and obesity. Diabetes, Metabolic Syndrome and Obesity: Targets and Therapy. 2012:5 175-189.

[19] Spreadbury, I. Comparison with ancestral diets suggests dense acellular carbohydrates promote an inflammatory microbiota, and may be the primary dietary cause of leptin resistance and obesity. Diabetes Metab Syndr Obes 2012, 5, 175-89.

[20] Hujoel, P. Dietary carbohydrates and dental systemic diseases. J Dent Res. 2009: 88(6), 490-502.

[21] Lockhart, PB, et al. Periodontal disease and atherosclerotic vascular disease: does the evidence support an independent association? Circulation. 2012 May 22;125(20):2520-44.

[22] Spreadbury, Ian. Comparison with ancestral diets suggests dense acellular carbohydrates promote an inflammatory microbiota, and may be the primary dietary cause of leptin resistance and obesity. Diabetes, Metabolic Syndrome and Obesity: Targets and Therapy. 2012:5 175-189.

[23] Baumgartner S, et al. The impact of the stoneage diet on gingival conditions in the absence of oral hygiene. J Perio, 2009:80 759-768.

[24] Mente, A; Razak, F; Blankenberg, S; et al. Ethnic variation in adiponectin and leptin levels and their association with adiposity and insulin resistance. Diabetes Care. 2010:33(7) 1629-1634.

[25] Genuis, Stephen. What's out there making us sick? J. Environmental and Public Health 2012 Article ID 605137.

[26] Bland, Jeffrey S. The Disease Delusion. Chapter 3 The Functional Medicine Revolution: Winning the Battle with Chronic Illness, 75-76. New York, Harper-Collins Publishers, 2014.

[27] Davis, Brenda. Defeating diabetes: a story of hope from the Marshall Islands. A seminar presented at the Food As Medicine conference. Indianapolis, IN. June 2013.

[28] Jonsson T, et al. Beneficial effects of a Paleolithic diet on cardiovascular risk factors in type 2 diabetes: a randomized cross-over pilot study. Cardiovase Diabetol. 2009;8:35.

[29] Frassetto, LA, et al. Metabolic and physiologic improvements from consuming a Paleolithic, hunter-gatherer type diet. Eur J Clin Hutr. 2009 Aug;63(8) 947-5.

[30] O'Dea K. Marked improvement in carbohydrate and lipid metabolism in diabetic Australian aborigines after temporary reversion to traditional lifestyle. Diabetes. 1984;33(6) 596-603.

[31] Spreadbury, Ian. Comparison with ancestral diets suggests dense acellular carbohydrates promote an inflammatory microbiota, and may be the primary dietary cause of leptin resistance and obesity. Diabetes, Metabolic Syndrome and Obesity: Targets and Therapy. 2012:5 175-189.

[32] Spreadbury, Ian. Comparison with ancestral diets suggests dense acellular carbohydrates promote an inflammatory microbiota, and may be the primary dietary cause of leptin resistance and obesity. Diabetes, Metabolic Syndrome and Obesity: Targets and Therapy. 2012:5 175-189.

[33] www.ndb.nal.usda.gov (homepage on Internet). NDL/FNIC Food Composition Database. Agricultural Research Service National Agricultural Library (modified Dec 7, 2011. Available from http://ndb.nal.usda.gov/ndb/foods. Accessed November 2014.

[34] www.ndb.nal.usda.gov (homepage on Internet). NDL/FNIC Food Composition Database. Agricultural Research Service National Agricultural Library (modified Dec 7, 2011. Available from http://ndb.nal.usda.gov. Accessed November 2014.

[35] http://www.ncbi.nlm.nih.gov/pubmed/19968914

[36] http://www.ncbi.nlm.nih.gov/pmc/articles/PMC3402009/

[37] http://ajcn.nutrition.or/content/71/3/665.full

[38] http://www.ncbi.nlm.nih.gov/pubmed/16421925

[39] http://www.ncbi.nlm.nih.gov/pmc/articles/PMC2684040/

[40]http://www.cdc.gov/breastfeeding/pdf/2014breastfeedingreportcard.pdf

[41] http://www.brianpalmerdds.com/bfeed_oralcavity.htm

[42] http://www.ncbi.nlm.nih.gov/pmc/articles/PMC3910336/

[43] http://www.ncbi.nlm.nih.gov/pmc/articles/PMC3809193/

[44] http://www.ncbi.nlm.nih.gov/pubmed/24880501

[45] http://www.ncbi.nlm.nih.gov/pubmed/22319749

[46] http://www.ncbi.nlm.nih.gov/pmc/articles/PMC4100321/

[47] http://www.ncbi.nlm.nih.gov/pmc/articles/PMC4114298/

[48] http://www.ncbi.nlm.nih.gov/pmc/articles/PMC3592792/

[49] http://www.ncbi.nlm.nih.gov/pmc/articles/PMC3925391/

[50] . http://www.ncbi.nlm.nih.gov/pubmed/25825113

[51] https://books.google.com/books?id=P_89d-5gzjUC&pg=PA109&lpg=PA109&dq=ebers+papyrus+and+bad+breath&source=bl&ots=kwT7vYC4ho&sig=hpmhU-LvsMTtuoJHmTDZT77TEhY&hl=en&sa=X&ei=8aGRVcqKM4m1-AHnyoHwBA&ved=0CCwQ6AEwAg#v=onepage&q=ebers%20papyrus%20and%20bad%20breath&f=false

[52] http://www.ncbi.nlm.nih.gov/pubmed/?term=krespi+yp+the+relationship+between+oral+malodor

[53] http://www.ncbi.nlm.nih.gov/pubmed/11493349

[54] http://www.ncbi.nlm.nih.gov/pmc/articles/PMC3925391/

[55] http://www.scielo.br/scielo.php?script=sci_arttext&pid=S1806-83242014000100228&lng=en&nrm=iso&tlng=en

[56] Eke, P.I.; Dye, B.A.; Wei, L.; Thornton-Evans, G.O.; Genco, R.J. Prevalence of Periodontitis in Adults in the United States: 2009 and 2010. JDR. 2012:10, 914-920.

[57] http://www.ncbi.nlm.nih.gov/pubmed/22826636

[58] http://scienceblog.com/40178/poor-sleep-quality-increases-inflammation-community-study-finds/#OdxOK7HPUX8L9iR1.99

[59] http://www.ncbi.nlm.nih.gov/pubmed/20036931

[60] http://www.ncbi.nlm.nih.gov/pubmed/25428651

[61] http://www.ncbi.nlm.nih.gov/pubmed/16840584

[62] http://www.ncbi.nlm.nih.gov/pubmed/25488896

[63] http://www.ncbi.nlm.nih.gov/pubmed/24161699

[64] Spreadbury, Ian. Comparison with ancestral diets suggests dense acellular carbohydrates promote an inflammatory microbiota, and may be the primary dietary cause of leptin resistance and obesity. Diabetes, Metabolic Syndrome and Obesity: Targets and Therapy. 2012:5 175-189.

[65] https://www.ncbi.nlm.nih.gov/pubmed/?term=antimicrobial+effects+of+essential+oils+in+humans Accessed on 12/28/16.

[66] http://www.oreganopro.com/oreganofaq.asp

[67] http://www.ncbi.nlm.nih.gov/pmc/articles/PMC4055614/

[68] http://physrev.physiology.org/content/91/1/151.long

[69] http://www.hopkinsarthritis.org/physician-corner/rheumatology-rounds/round-34-periodontal-disease-and-rheumatoid-arthritis/

[70] http://www.ncbi.nlm.nih.gov/pmc/articles/PMC3816614/

[71] Bianconi, E; Piovesan, A; Facchin, F; et al. An estimation of the number of cells in the human body. Ann Hum Biol. 2013; Nov-Dec 40(6) 463-471.

[72] Lichtenstein, P, et al. Environmental and heritable factors in the causation of cancer – analyses of cohorts of twins from Sweden, Denmark, and Finland. N Engl J Med. 2000 Jul 13:243(2) 78-85.

[73] Genuis, Stephen. What's out there making us sick? J. Environmental and Public Health 2012 Article ID 605137.

[74] Alberts, B; Johnson, A; Lewis, J; Raff, M Roberts, K; Walter, P. Molecular Biology of the Cell 4th ed. NY, Garland Publishing 2002.

[75] https://www.collegeofintegrativemedicine.org/

[76] https://www.functionalmedicine.org/

[77] http://www.functionalmedicineuniversity.com/

[78] Gershon, Michael. The second brain: a groundbreaking new understanding of nervous disorders of the stomach and intestine. New York, HarperCollins Publishers, 1998.

[79] Frank, DN, et al. Molecular-phylogenetic characterization of microbial community imbalances in human inflammatory bowel diseases. Proc Natl Acad Sci USA. 2007; 104: 13780–13785.

[80] Braniste, V; et al. The gut microbiota influences blood-brain barrier permeability in mice. Sci Transl Med. 2014; 6, 263ra158.

[81] Anaerobic bacteria can survive without oxygen in the large intestine. These special bacteria are responsible for metabolizing carbohydrates and proteins, which are converted into short-chain fatty acids (especially butyric acid). The cells of the colon (called colonocytes) are nourished by these short-chain fatty acids.

[82] These are some of the byproducts of healthy bacteria that help the liver regulate blood sugar (glucose) metabolism.

[83] Healthy bacteria improve the absorption of micronutrients such as calcium, magnesium, iron, and vitamin D by fermenting carbohydrates in our guts.

[84] Healthy bacteria synthesize biotin (vitamin B7), folate, and other B vitamins as well as vitamins K and E.

[85] Intestinal microbes convert these substances into other useful end products.

[86] Gut bacteria assist the cell lining of the gut to function and reproduce properly.

[87] Immune cells live throughout the digestive tract where about 70% of the body's immune system resides. A healthy gut microbiome assists the immune cells to defend themselves from invaders.

[88] Fasano, A. Zonulin and Its Regulation of Intestinal Barrier Function: The Biological Door to Inflammation, Autoimmunity, and Cancer. Physiological Reviews Published. 2011 Vol. 91 no. 1, 151-175

[89] Paleo diet = lean meat, fish, fruits, vegetables, root vegetables, eggs, nuts

[90] Mediterranean diet = whole grains, low-fat dairy products, vegetables, fruits, fish, oil, margarine

[91] Diabetes diet = majority of energy would come from vegetables, root vegetables, dietary fiber, whole grain bread, whole grain cereal, fruits, berries, with decreased amounts of total fat

[92] Lindeberg, S; et al. A Paleolithic diet improves glucose tolerance more than a Mediterranean-like diet in individuals with ischaemic heart disease. Diabetologia. 2007 Sep;50(9):1795-807.

[93] Osterdahl, M; et al. Effects of a short-term intervention with a Paleolithic diet in healthy volunteers. Eur J Clin Nutr. 2008 May;62(5):682-5.

[94] Jönsson, T; et al. Beneficial effects of a Paleolithic diet on cardiovascular risk factors in type 2 diabetes: a randomized crossover pilot study. Cardiovasc Diabetol. 2009; 8: 35.

[95] Jönsson, T; et al. A Paleolithic diet is more satiating per calorie than a Mediterranean-like diet in individuals with ischemic heart disease. Nutr Metab (Lond). 2010; 7: 85.

[96] Frassetto, LA; et al. Metabolic and physiologic improvements from consuming a Paleolithic, hunter-gatherer type diet. Eur J Clin Nutr. 2009 Aug;63(8):947-55.

[97] Ryberg, M; et al. A Paleolithic-type diet causes strong tissue-specific effects on ectopic fat deposition in obese postmenopausal women. J Intern Med. 2013 Jul;274(1):67-76.

[98] Mellberg, C; et al. Long-term effects of a Paleolithic-type diet in obese postmenopausal women: a two-year randomized trial. Eur J Clin Nutr. 2014 Mar; 68(3): 350–357.

[99] Boers, I; et al. Favourable effects of consuming a Paleolithic-type diet on characteristics of the metabolic syndrome: a randomized controlled pilot-study. Lipids Health Dis. 2014; 13(1): 160.

[100] Metabolic Syndrome characteristics = increased body weight, increased waist circumference, increased blood pressure, increased triglycerides, decreased HDL cholesterol, increased insulin resistance, increased fasting blood glucose

[101] Dutch Healthy Reference diet = similar to the Mediterranean diet and the Diabetes diet

[102] Freeman, H. Celiac Disease: A Disorder Emerging from Antiquity, Its Evolving Classification and Risk, and Potential New Treatment Paradigms. Gut Liver. 2015 Jan; 9(1): 28–37.

[103] Lindeberg, S; Lundh, B. Apparent absence of stroke and ischaemic heart disease in a traditional Melanesian island: a clinical study in Kitava. J Intern Med. 1993; 233(3): 269-275.

[104] Johnson, A; Dehrens, C. Nutritional criteria in Machiguenga food production decisions: a linear-programming analysis. Hum Ecl. 1982; 10(2): 167-189.

[105] Biss, K; et al. Some unique biologic characteristics of the Masai of East Africa. N Engl J Med. 1971; 284(13): 694-699.

[106] Truswell, AS; et al. Blood pressures of !Kung bushmen in Northern Botswania. Am Heart J. 1972;83(1):5-12.

[107] Schulz, LO; et al. Effects of traditional and western environments on prevalence of type 2 diabetes in Pima Indians in Mexico and the US. Diabetes Care. 2006; 29(8): 1866-1871.

[108] Ibid.

[109] London, DS; Beezhold, B. A phytochemical-rich diet may explain the absence of age-related decline in visual acuity of Amazonian hunter-gatherers in Ecuador. Nutr Res. 2015 Feb;35(2):107-17.

[110] Cornier MA, Dabelea D, Hernandez TL, Lindstrom RC, Steig AJ, Stob NR, van Pet RE, Wang H, Eckel RH. The metabolic syndrome. Endocr Rev. 2008;29(7):777–822. doi: 10.1210/er.2008-0024. [PubMed]

[111] Grundy SM. Metabolic syndrome: connecting and reconciling cardiovascular and diabetes worlds. J Am Coll Cardiol. 2006;47(6):1093–1100. doi: 10.1016/j.jacc.2005.11.046. [PubMed]

[112] Ford ES, Li C, Sattar N. Metabolic syndrome and incident diabetes: current state of evidence. Diabetes Care. 2008;31:1898–1904. doi: 10.2337/dc08-0423. [PMC free article] [PubMed]

[113] Gami AS, Witt BJ, Howard DE, Erwin PJ, Gami LA, Somers VK, Montori VM. Metabolic syndrome and risk of incident cardiovascular events and death: a systematic review and meta-analyses of longitudinal studies. J Am Coll Cardiol. 2007;49:403–414. doi: 10.1016/j.jacc.2006.09.032. [PubMed]

[114] Ruiz-Núñez B, Pruimboom L, Dijck-Brouwer DA, Muskiet FA. Lifestyle and nutritional imbalances associated with Western diseases: causes and consequences of chronic systemic low-grade inflammation in an evolutionary context. J Nutr Biochem. 2013;24(7):1183–1201. doi: 10.1016/j.jnutbio.2013.02.009. [PubMed]

[115] Cordain L, Eaton S, Sebastian A. Origins and evolution of the western diet Health implications for the 21st century. Am J Clin Nutr. 2005;81:341–354. [PubMed]

[116] Eaton SB, Cordain L. Evolutionary aspects of diet: old genes, new fuels. Nutritional changes since agriculture. World Rev Nutr Diet. 1997;81:26–37. doi: 10.1159/000059599. [PubMed]

[117] Eaton SB, Eaton SB., III Paleolithic vs modern diets-selected pathophysiological implications. Eur J Nutr. 2000;39:67–70. doi: 10.1007/s003940070032. [PubMed]

[118] Jansson B. Dietary, total body and intracellular potassium-to-sodium ratios and their influence on cancer. Cancer Detect Prev. 1990;14:563–565. [PubMed]

[119] Mann JI, De Leeuw I, Hermansen K, Karamanos B, Karlström B, Katsilambros N, Riccardi G, Rivellese AA, Rizkalla S, Slama G, Toeller M, Uusitupa M, Vessby B, Diabetes and Nutrition Study Group (DNSG) of the European Association Evidence-based nutritional approaches to the treatment and prevention of diabetes mellitus. Nutr Metab Cardiovasc Dis. 2004;14(6):373–394. doi: 10.1016/S0939-4753(04)80028-0. [PubMed]

[120] O'Keefe JH, Jr, Cordain L. Cardiovascular disease resulting from a diet and lifestyle at odds with our Paleolithic genome: how to become a 21st-century hunter-gatherer. Mayo Clin Proc. 2004;79:101–108. doi: 10.4065/79.1.101. [PubMed]

[121] Sebastian A, Frassetto LA, Sellmeyer DE, Merriam RL, Morris RC., Jr Estimation of the net acid load of the diet of ancestral preagricultural Homo sapiens and their hominid ancestors. Am J Clin Nutr. 2002;76:1308–1316. [PubMed]

[122] Sebastian A, Frassetto LA, Sellmeyer DE, Morris RC., Jr The evolution-informed optimal dietary potassium intake of human beings greatly exceeds current and recommended intakes. Semin Nephrol. 2006;26(6):447–453. doi: 10.1016/j.semnephrol.2006.10.003. [PubMed]

[123] Osterdahl M, Kocturk T, Koochek A, Wändell PE. Effects of a short-term intervention with a Paleolithic diet in healthy volunteers. Eur J Clin Nutr. 2008;62(5):682–685. doi: 10.1038/sj.ejcn.1602790. [PubMed]

[124] Ryberg M, Sandberg S, Mellberg C, Stegle O, Lindahl B, Larsson C, Hauksson J, Olsson T. A Paleolithic-type diet causes strong tissue-specific effects on ectopic fat deposition in obese postmenopausal women. J Int Med. 2013;274(1):67–76. doi: 10.1111/joim.12048. [PubMed]

[125] Frasetto LA, Schloetter M, Mietus-Synder M, Morris RC, Jr, Sebastian A. Metabolic and physiologic improvement from

consuming a Paleolithic, hunter-gatherer type diet. Eur J Clin Nutr. 2009;63(8):947–955. doi: 10.1038/ejcn.2009.4. [PubMed]

[126] (Boers, I; et al. Favourable effects of consuming a Paleolithic-type diet on characteristics of the metabolic syndrome: a randomized controlled pilot-study. Lipids Health Dis. 2014; 13(1): 160.)

[127] http://www.ncbi.nlm.nih.gov/pubmed/?term=Circulation+1997%3B96%3A2520-2525

[128] http://www.webmd.com/diet/phytonutrients-faq (homepage on Internet). Accessed on 11/25/2014.

[129] Cordain L, Miller JB, Eaton SB, Mann N, Holt SH, Speth JD. Plant-animal subsistence ratios and macronutrient energy estimations in worldwide hunter-gatherer diets. Am J Clin Nutr. 2000 Mar;71(3):682-92.

[130] O'Keefe JH, Cordain L. Cardiovascular disease resulting from a diet and lifestyle at odds with our Paleolithic genome: how to become a 21st-century hunter-gatherer. Mayo Clin. Proc. 2004;79(1):101-8.

[131] Eaton SB, Konner MJ. Review Paleolithic nutrition revisited: A twelve-year retrospective on its nature and implications. Eur. J. Clin. Nutr. 1997;51(4):207-216.

[132] http://www.ncbi.nlm.nih.gov/pmc/articles/PMC4006742/

[133] http://www.ncbi.nlm.nih.gov/pmc/articles/PMC4326908/

[134] Chowdhury R, Warnakula S, Kunutsor S, et al. Association of dietary, circulating, and supplement fatty acids with coronary risk: a systematic review and meta-analysis. Ann Intern Med., 2014: Mar 18;160(6):398-406.

[135] http://nutritiondata.self.com (homepage on Internet). Accessed on 12/24/2014.

[136] Białek, A; Teryks, M,; Tokarz A. Conjugated linolenic acids (CLnA, super CLA) - natural sources and biological activity. Postepy Hig Med Dosw (Online). 2014 Nov 6;68(0):1238-50.

[137] Chapman, V. J., and D. J. Chapman. Sea vegetables (algae as food for man). *Seaweeds and their Uses.* Springer Netherlands (1980): 62-97.

[138] Romarís–Hortas, Vanessa, et al. Bioavailability study using an in-vitro method of iodine and bromine in edible seaweed. Food Chemistry. 2011; 124.4: 1747-1752.

[139] Prasad, Divyashree and Kunnaiah, Ravi. *Punica granatum*: A review on its potential role in treating periodontal disease. J Indian Soc Periodontol. 2014 Jul-Aug; 18(4): 428–432.

[140] Sangeetha J, Vijayalakshmi K. Antimicrobial activity of rind extracts of Punica granatum Linn. The Bioscan. 2011;6:119–124.

[141] Pereira JV, Pereira MDSV, Higino JS, Sampio FC, Alves PM, Araujo CRF. Studies with the extract of the Punica granatum Linn.(Pomegranate): Antimicrobial effect "in vitro" and clinical evaluation of a toothpaste upon microorganisms of the oral biofilm. Journal of Dental Science. 2005;20:262–269.

[142] Sastravaha G, Yotnuengnit P, Booncong P, Sangtherapitikul P. Adjunctive periodontal treatment with *Centella asiatica* and *Punica granatum* extracts. A preliminary study. J Int Acad Periodontol. 2003;5:106–115.

[143] Badria FA, Zidan OA. Natural products for dental caries prevention. J Med Food. 2004;7:381–384.

[144] DiSilvestro RA, DiSilvestro DJ, DiSilvestro DJ. Pomegranate extract mouth rinsing effects on saliva measures relevant to gingivitis risk. Phytother Res. 2009;23:1123–1127.

[145] Ahuja S, Dodwad V, Kukreja BJ, Mehra P, Kukreja P. A comparative evaluation of efficacy of Punica granatum and

chlorhexidine on plaque and gingivitis. J Int Clin Dent Res Organ. 2011;3:29–32.

[146] Menezes SM, Cordeiro LN, Viana GS. *Punica granatum* (pomegranate) extract is active against dental plaque. J Herb Pharmacother. 2006;6:79–92.

[147] Dye BA, Kruszon-Moran D, McQuillan G. The relationship between periodontal disease attributes and *Helicobacter pylori* infection among adults in the United States. Am J Public Health. 2002;92:1809–1815.

[148] Umeda M, Kobayashi H, Takeuchi Y, Hayashi J, Morotome-Hayashi Y, Yano K, et al. High prevalence of *Helicobacter pylori* detected by PCR in the oral cavities of periodontitis patients. J Periodontol. 2003;74:129–134.

[149] Gebara EC, Pannuti C, Faria CM, Chehter L, Mayer MP, Lima LA. Prevalence of *Helicobacter pylori* detected by polymerase chain reaction in the oral cavity of periodontitis patients. Oral Microbiol Immunol. 2004;19:277–280.

[150] Riggio MP, Lennon A. Identification by PCR of *Helicobacter pylori* in subgingival plaque of adult periodontitis patients. J Med Microbiol. 1999;48:317–322.

[151] Hajimahmoodi M, Shams-Ardakani M, Saniee P, Siavoshi F, Mehrabani M, Hosseinzadeh H, et al. *In vitro* antibacterial activity of some Iranian medicinal plant extracts against *Helicobacter pylori*. Nat Prod Res. 2011;25:1059–1066.

[152] Howell AB, D'Souza DH. The Pomegranate: Effects on bacteria and viruses that influence human health. Evid Based Complement Alternat Med 2013. 2013:606212.

[153] Stamatova I, Meurman JH. Probiotics and periodontal disease. Periodontol 2000. 2009;51:141–151.

[154] Prakash CVS, Prakash I. Bioactive Chemical Constituents from Pomegranate (*Punica granatum*) Juice, Seed and Peel-A Review. Int J Res Chem Environ. 2011;1:1–18.

[155] Abdollahzdeh SH, Mashouf R, Mortazavi H, Moghaddam M, Roozbahani N, Vahedi M. Antibacterial and Antifungal activities of *Punica granatum* Peel extracts against Oral Pathogens. J Dent (Tehran) 2011;8:1–6.

[156] Koh KH, Tham FY. Screening of traditional Chinese medicinal plants for quorum-sensing inhibitors activity. J Microbiol Immunol Infect. 2011;44:144–148.

[157] Abdollahzdeh SH, Mashouf R, Mortazavi H, Moghaddam M, Roozbahani N, Vahedi M. Antibacterial and Antifungal activities of *Punica granatum* Peel extracts against Oral Pathogens. J Dent (Tehran) 2011;8:1–6.

[158] Naqvi S, Khan MSY, Vohora SB. Anti-bacterial, anti-fungal and anthelmintic investigations on Indian medicinal plants. Fitoterapia. 1991;62:221–228.

[159] Miguel MG, Neves MA, Antunes MD. Pomegranate (*Punica granatum* L.): A medicinal plant with myriad biologic properties: A short review. J Med Plants Res. 2010;4:2836–2847.

[160] https://www.youtube.com/watch?v=sHyqoeB0Wlk

[161] http://www.ncbi.nlm.nih.gov/pmc/articles/PMC3583289/

[162] http://www.ncbi.nlm.nih.gov/pubmed/12935325

[163] http://www.woundsresearch.com/article/honey-biologic-wound-dressing

[164] http://www.ncbi.nlm.nih.gov/pubmed/18454257

[165] http://www.ncbi.nlm.nih.gov/pubmed/25226738

[166] http://www.ncbi.nlm.nih.gov/pmc/articles/PMC3909917/

[167] http://www.ncbi.nlm.nih.gov/pubmed/15117561

[168] http://www.ncbi.nlm.nih.gov/pmc/articles/PMC4095052/

[169] http://www.ncbi.nlm.nih.gov/pubmed/10784339

[170] http://www.ncbi.nlm.nih.gov/pubmed/19155427

[171] http://www.ncbi.nlm.nih.gov/pubmed/12617614

[172] http://nutritiondata.self.com (homepage on Internet). Accessed on 12/24/2014.

[173] Aggarwal, Bharat; Yost, Debora. Healing Spices. New York, Sterling Publishing, 2011.

[174] http://articles.mercola.com/sites/articles/archive/2011/07/31/dr-natasha-campbell-mcbride-on-gaps-nutritional-program.aspx

[175] Antonoglou, GN; Knuuttila M; et al. Low serum level of 1,25(OH)2 D is associated with chronic periodontitis. J Periodontal Res. 2014 Jul 7. doi: 10.1111/jre.12207. [Epub ahead of print]

[176] Anand, N; Chandrasekaran, SC; et al. Vitamin D and periodontal health: Current concepts. J Indian Soc Periodontol. 2013 May-Jun; 17(3): 302–308.

[177] Forrest KY, Stuhldreher WL. Prevalence and correlates of vitamin D deficiency in US adults. Nutr Res. 2011 Jan;31(1):48-54.

[178] Bischoff-Ferrari, HA. Optimal serum 25-hydroxyvitamin D levels for multiple health outcomes. Adv Exp Med Biol. 2008;624:55-71.

[179] Heaney, RP; Armas, LAG. Quantifying the vitamin D economy. Nutrition Reviews. 2015; 73(1); 51-67.

[180] Alshouibi, EN; Kaye, EK; et al. Vitamin D and Periodontal Health in Older Menl. J Dent Res. Aug 2013; 92(8): 689–693.

[181] Martelli, SM; Martelli, M; et al. Vitamin D: relevance in dental practice. Clin Cases Miner Bone Metab. 2014 Jan-Apr; 11(1): 15–19.

[182] Andrukhov, O; Andrukhova, O; et al. Both 25-Hydroxyvitamin-D_3 and 1,25-Dihydroxyvitamin-D_3 Reduces Inflammatory Response in Human Periodontal Ligament Cells. PLoS One. 2014; 9(2): e90301. Published online Feb 28, 2014. doi: 10.1371/journal.pone.0090301 PMCID: PMC3938673

[183] http://dminder.ontometrics.com/

[184] Cordain L. The nutritional characteristics of a contemporary diet based upon Paleolithic food groups. J Am Neutraceut Assoc 2002; 5:15-24.

[185] http://www.greenpasture.org/public/Products/ButterCodLiverBl end/index.cfm

[186] http://www.oregonswildharvest.com/owh/browse/product/kelp

[187] http://www.prescript-assist.com/

[188] http://www.ncbi.nlm.nih.gov/pmc/articles/PMC3292009/

[189] http://drdanenberg.com/nrf2-is-not-a-new-password/

[190] Akande, K.E., Doma, U.D., Agu, H.O., and Adamu H.M. Major antinutrients found in plant protein sources: their effect on nutrition. Pakistan Journal of Nutrition. 2010; 9 (8): 827-832

[191] Suez, J; Korem, T; et al. Artificial sweeteners induce glucose intolerance by altering the gut microbiota. Nature. 2014 Oct 9;514(7521):181-6

[192] Swithers. SE. Artificial sweeteners produce the counterintuitive effect of inducing metabolic derangements. Trends in Endocrinology and Metabolism. 2013. 1–11

[193] http://www.sciencedirect.com/science/article/pii/S0166432814008 50X#bib0725

[194] http://www.ncbi.nlm.nih.gov/pmc/articles/PMC3666060/

[195] http://www.ncbi.nlm.nih.gov/pmc/articles/PMC4075302/

[196] http://www.ncbi.nlm.nih.gov/pmc/articles/PMC3895311/

[197] http://www.ncbi.nlm.nih.gov/pmc/articles/PMC3666060/

[198] http://www.ncbi.nlm.nih.gov/pmc/articles/PMC4211166/

[199] http://www.ncbi.nlm.nih.gov/pmc/articles/PMC4147812/

[200] http://www.bengreenfieldfitness.com/2011/07/top-10-reasons-exercise-is-bad-for-you

[201] www.ccrlab.com, 719-550-0008

[202] www.biocomplabs.com, 800-331-2303

[203] www.melisa.org

[204] http://www.ncbi.nlm.nih.gov/pubmed/?term=Effect+of+oil+gum+massage+therapy+on+common+pathogenic+oral+microorganisms+-+A+randomized+controlled+trial

[205] http://www.usa.philips.com/e/ohc/consumer/cons-range-toothbrushes.html

[206] http://www.oralb.com/products/electric-toothbrush

[207] www.GumBrand.com

[208] http://www.ncbi.nlm.nih.gov/pubmed/24165218

[209] http://dminder.ontometrics.com/

[210] http://www.ncbi.nlm.nih.gov/pmc/articles/PMC4518639/

[211] http://www.trikke.com

[212] http://www.pullupbarss.com

[213] https://www.youtube.com/watch?v=76HjVOoUX6U

[214] https://www.youtube.com/watch?v=UayvOd0xlAU

[215] https://www.youtube.com/watch?v=HNRiFnyqTxQ

[216] https://www.youtube.com/watch?v=GrHG7m4m4-A

[217] http://www.nordictrack.com/fitness/en/NordicTrack/Skiers/nordictrack-classic-pro-skier?utm_source=Shopzilla&utm_medium=cpc

[218] http://www.pedometerreviewsdepot.com

[219] http://www.nextavenue.org/article/2014-10/health-hazards-sitting-too-much

[220] http://www.youtube.com/watch?v=JyVXWH87jXo

[221] http://fitness.mercola.com/sites/fitness/archive/2013/12/20/intermittent-fasting-weight-loss.aspx

[222] http://wellness.mcmaster.ca/resources/relaxation/musclerelation.html

[223] http://www.plosone.org/article/fetchArticle.action?articleURI=info%3Adoi%2F10.1371%2Fjournal.pone.0000698

[224] http://www.localharvest.org/csa

[225] www.vitamix.com

[226] https://www.nutribulletrx.com

[227] http://www.eufic.org/article/en/nutrition/nutrigenomics/artid/nutrition-human-genome-2/

[228] http://nutrigenomics.ucdavis.edu/?page=information

[229] www.amrapnutrition.com

[230] http://www.gapsdiet.com/

[231] http://www.marksdailyapple.com/remember-the-80-20-principle/#axzz3NNtdIYck

[232] http://thepaleodiet.com/the-atlanta-journal-constitution-qa-with-dr-cordain

[233] http://suppversity.blogspot.com/2014/11/calorie-shifting-refeeding-for-max-fat.html

[234] http://www.ncbi.nlm.nih.gov/pubmed/20685357

[235] http://www.ncbi.nlm.nih.gov/pubmed/15925707

[236] http://www.ncbi.nlm.nih.gov/pubmed/18937164?ordinalpos=1&itool=EntrezSystem2.PEntrez.Pubmed.Pubmed_ResultsPanel.Pubmed_DiscoveryPanel.Pubmed_Discovery_RA&linkpos=5&log$=relatedreviews&logdbfrom=pubmed

[237] http://www.ncbi.nlm.nih.gov/pubmed/23954367

[238] http://www.plosone.org/article/info%3Adoi%2F10.1371%2Fjournal.pone.0004377

[239] www.vitamix.com

[240] https://www.nutribulletrx.com

[241] Tam, M; Fong, H. Nom Nom Paleo: Food for Humans. 2013. Andrews McMeed Publishing, MO.

[242] https://www.bulletproofexec.com/bulletproof-coffee-recipe

[243] https://www.drfuhrman.com/library/choosing_the_right_cinnamon.aspx

[244] www.matchasource.com

[245] http://civilizedcavemancooking.com/recipes/desserts/paleo-banana-bread/

[246] http://paleopumpkinmuffins.com/

[247] http://paleoleap.com/flourless-brownies/

[248] http://www.janssushibar.com/french-onion-oxtail-stew/

[249] Child, J; Bertholle, L; Beck, S. *Mastering the art of French cooking.* Alfred A. Knopf, Inc., New York, 1961, p 43.

[250] http://www.thepaleomom.com/2012/09/perfect-paleo-pancakes.html

[251] Joulwain, M. Well Fed. 2011. Smudge Publishing, TX.

CPSIA information can be obtained
at www.ICGtesting.com
Printed in the USA
LVHW030735051119
636371LV00004B/92/P

9 780999 157312